About the authors

DR AXEL KROEGER is a physician in Internal Medicine as well as Tropical Medicine. Following his work as a doctor for four years in the Amazonian area of Ecuador in the early 1970s, he worked for some years in a general hospital in Hamburg, following which he did a Master's Degree in Community Health at the London School of Hygiene and Tropical Medicine. In 1983 he was appointed Professor of Tropical Medicine and Public Health at the University of Heidelburg. In 1993, he became Professor of International Community Health and Director of the Latin America Centre at the Liverpool School of Tropical Medicine in the United Kingdom.

REGINA GÖRGEN is a health educationalist at the Institute of Tropical Hygiene and Public Health, University of Heidelburg. As a consultant in various African countries as well as Uzbekistan, she has worked on communications between service providers and users in family planning and AIDS prevention.

SONIA JANETH DIAZ MONSALVE specializes in health management, health planning, and the implementation and evaluation of health programmes. From 1985 to 1990 she was Director, School of Nursing, Cucuta, Colombia. She then taught at the Liverpool School of Tropical Medicine, after which she returned to her lecturing post in Colombia. She was appointed Lecturer in Health Management in the Faculty of Health Sciences, Universidad Francisco de Paula Santander, Cucuta, Colombia in 1995.

CARLOS MONTOYA AGUILAR is a medical doctor and pediatrician. In 1969 he became Professor of Medical Care and Health Planning at the University of Chile. In 1973, he left the country and was appointed to the staff of WHO in Geneva where he served sixteen years in various capacities before returning to his home country in 1991 where he became National Coordinator of the Equity Approach in Health at the Ministry of Health. He is the author of more than 100 publications in the fields of public health and paediatrics which have been published in both national and international journals.

WOLFGANG BICHMANN is a specialist in international community health, as well as tropical and environmental health issues. He has had extensive practical experience since 1979 in both West Africa and South Asia. Since 1983 he has taught at the Institute of Tropical Hygiene and Public Health at Heidelberg University. He is currently a Senior Public Health Advisor to the German Development Bank, as well as serving as a member of WHO's Forum on Health Sector Reform and on the Editorial Advisory Committee of the Alternative Health Resources and Teaching Aids Group's (AHRTAG) Health Action Newsletter.

TRAINING MANUALS

THE USE OF
Epidemiology
IN LOCAL HEALTH PLANNING

A TRAINING MANUAL

AXEL KROEGER • CARLOS MONTOYA-AGUILAR

WOLFGANG BICHMANN • REGINA GÖRGEN

SONIA JANETH DIAZ

NPPHCN

NATIONAL PROGRESSIVE PRIMARY
HEALTH CARE NETWORK

South Africa

The Use of Epidemiology in Local Health Planning: A Training Manual was published in 1997 by
Zed Books Ltd, 7 Cynthia Street, London N1 9JF and 165 First Avenue, Atlantic Highlands, New
Jersey, 01776, and in Southern Africa by National Progressive Primary Health Care Network (NPPHCN),
PO Box 32095, Braamfontein 2017, Gauteng.

Revised and updated from the Spanish edition published in 1994 by Organización Panamericana de la Salud,
Oficina Sanitaria Panamericana, Oficina Regional de la Organización Mundial de la Salud under the title
*Materiales de Enseñanza sobre el Uso de la Epidemiología en la Programación de Los Servicios locales de
Salud (SILOS)*.

The Federal Republic of Germany through the Public Health Promotion Centre of the German Foundation for
International Development has contributed to the production of this publication with DM16,000 in order to reduce
the price for individual copies and make them accessible to a larger number of users, especially in the South.

Copyright © Axel Kroeger, Carlos Montoya-Aguilar, Wolfgang Bichmann, Regina Görgen,
         Sonia Janeth Diaz 1997

Cover design by Andrew Corbett
Typeset by Nicola Meneses
Visuals and design by A. Kroeger, N. Meneses, and L. Kraus (drawings)
Printed and bound in the United Kingdom by Biddles Ltd, Guildford and King's Lynn

A catalogue record for this book is available from the British Library

Library of Congress Cataloging-in-Publication Data

The use of epidemiology in local health planning: a training manual/Axel Kroeger...[et al]
p. cm
Includes bibliographical references and index
ISBN 1-85649-481-0 (cloth).   ISBN 1-85649-482-9 (pbk).
1. Epidemiology. 2. Community health services – planning 3. Community health aides. I. Kroeger, Axel
[DNLM: 1. Community Health Planning – methods. 2. Epidemiology. WA 546. 1 U84 1997]
RA652. U84 1997
614. 4 – dc20
DNLM/DLC for Library of Congress   96-36126
                                                                              CIP

ISBN 1 85649 481 0 hb ✓
ISBN 1 85649 482 9 pb

Southern Africa
ISBN 0 620 21089 3 pb

CONTENTS

Preface   ix

Introduction   1
Why we wrote this book   1
How to use the materials   3
Organizing a workshop   10
Learning objectives of the training course   11
Basic assumptions for the success of the workshop   11

**PART A: WORKSHOP ON THE USE OF EPIDEMIOLOGY AT DISTRICT   13
            AND LOCAL LEVEL**

Schedule   15
Structure of the workshop   16

Module A1. The Nine Epidemiological Questions   18

Module A2. Exercises with Epidemiological Tools   23
1. What are the main health problems in your community?   23
2. How many cases or health events did you come across?   24
3. When do the cases or events generally occur?   26
4. Where do the cases or health events occur?   29
5. Who is affected?   30
6. Why does the problem occur?   33
7. What kind of measures did you yourself or others in the community take to cope with the problem?   35
8. What results have been achieved? What kind of difficulties did you encounter in trying to deal with   35
    the problem?
9. What else could be done? What kind of assistance is needed?   36

Module A3. Training in Epidemiological Thinking   39

Module A4. Who is affected? (The Risk Approach)   42

Module A5. An Epidemic Outbreak   44

PART B: ANALYSIS OF HEALTH SERVICES AND LOCAL PLANNING   49

Preparation and schedule of the workshop   51
Structure of the workshop on local programming   53

Module B1. Analysis of Health Services Problems   54

Module B2. Introduction to the Planning Matrix   65

Module B3. Improving Technical Work at Local Level   71

Module B4. Assessing the Quality of Services   76

Module B5. Improving Acceptance through Recognition of Local Cultural Factors   78

Module B6. Making a Census   80

Appendices

A.1. Pictures of Part A (to be cut out)   87
A.2. Possible Solutions to Exercises in Part A   111
A.3. Didactic Games and Questions Bank   119
A.4. Causation Tree (simplified)   129
B.1. Assessing Health Systems by Means of Indicators   131
B.2. Possible Solutions to Exercises in Part B   143
B.3. Didactic Games, Objectives, Targets and Indicators   149
B.4. Comparative Data from World Health Statistics   155
B.5. Exercise on Use of Indicators in Assessing Health Services   159

Bibliography   **165**

PREFACE

This book is about the 'democratization' of epidemiology and planning, bringing together the usefulness of epidemiological techniques and the practicality of planning tools down to local health services. The local team of health managers will be empowered to base their planning on a sound analysis of the health problems and the problems of the health services in their districts and communities. The educational approach described in this manual is a dynamic and participatory one; it overcomes one-way classroom teaching and uses problem-orientated training with emphasis on the interaction between facilitators and trainees and amongst the trainees themselves. In order to enhance the exchange of experiences a variety of training tools are used which also make the learning procedure pleasant without losing the path towards the general objective: to introduce participants to rational health planning on the basis of a detailed diagnosis of the local situation. The text is mainly designed for local health services and uses very few numbers and percentages; however it can easily be enriched by more sophisticated topics and materials which make it useful for postgraduate training in public health and international community health. The book has successfully been tested and used in Africa, Asia, Latin America and in European courses of postgraduate training.

A Note on Terminology: The terms used in referring to local-level health workers, who are the ultimate users of this book, vary from country to country. We have chosen to use the term Village Health Worker (VHW), but it should be seen as referring to Community Health Worker (CHW) and other equivalent roles, whatever their designation in particular countries may be.

INTRODUCTION

Why We Wrote This Book

The need for this kind of learning material

Developing epidemiological thinking among health workers is a long–term endeavour, which begins with their training, and should extend throughout their entire working life. It remains a challenge for professional epidemiologists to adapt their materials to the specific requirements of their respective target groups.

Although a number of books and various publications targeted at the district level health manager exist (e.g. McCuster 1982, McMahon et al. 1980, Kroeger and Luna 1992, Amonoo–Larzon et al. 1984, Vaughan and Morrow 1990, Annet and Cassels 1990), there is as yet no compilation of learning materials that could be used for the training of local health personnel in basic epidemiological thinking, community-health orientation and local planning. We used WHO Offset Publication No 70, 'The use of epidemiology in local health work,' and a report on its practical applications as the basis for our manual as well as previous experiences obtained in the Latin American Workshop for Applied Epidemiology for Health Services (TLEA) (Alarcón and Kroeger 1991).

The learning materials presented here are designed for local health workers and are meant to enhance the quality of their work by strengthening their analytical thinking and their understanding of reality at the local level in order to make better decisions and plans. Case studies from all over the world (WHO 1982) have shown health workers to be extremely knowledgeable about the health conditions prevailing in their respective communities. But as a result of their training, they have become mere followers of rules and regulations, shying away from a personal analysis of the health conditions in their own communities.

The health workers' dilemma

Although their tasks are to a great extent regulated by norms, health workers have a certain degree of freedom and sometimes even an obligation to analyse for themselves the health conditions in their own communities. The opportunities to make health plans are growing in the context of health sector reforms and decentralization. The present training materials are meant to motivate health workers to make use of their own sources of information at community level. The health workers' assessment of community-health problems should not be isolated from their other activities but become an integral part of them. It is important to strike the right balance between time spent on 'community diagnosis' and on the subsequent interventions. It may very well be that a health worker, who has come to regard epidemiology as an exciting new field of endeavour, will choose to spend much of his/her time on data collection and so neglect working on the results of the analysis. On the other hand, they may also have become so engrossed in a purely interventionist approach that they lose sight of the overall situation in the target population. Supervisors should advise their health personnel of the need to achieve an equilibrium between the two extremes.

Diagram 1

Two approaches of approximation

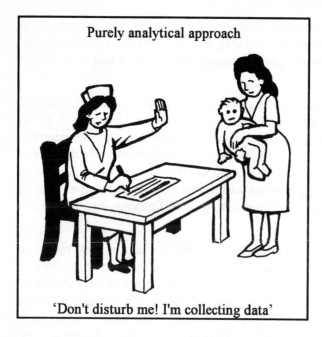

Purely analytical approach

'Don't disturb me! I'm collecting data'

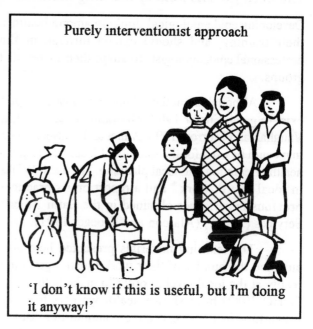

Purely interventionist approach

'I don't know if this is useful, but I'm doing it anyway!'

The need for adapting learning materials to the local situation

Although we do not doubt local health workers' ability to analyse health problems and their causes in a rational way, we hold the view that they do not necessarily think in the same manner and along the same lines as academically trained health managers. For instance, in many places they do not use maps for orientation; they generally do not employ percentages and means to express phenomena in numbers; they neither relate nor extrapolate particular health events to the whole of the population or to certain population groups, and so on.

But it is debatable whether people in general (and more particularly in this case, health workers who are gifted with an innate sense of orientation) should learn to use maps and numbers to express the frequency and importance of events, when they can achieve this in other ways. Should they learn about statistical population data to interpret and extrapolate epidemiological phenomena correctly if they can do so by other methods?

Adapting the learning materials as much as possible to the existing knowledge and skills of the local health workers thus takes on added importance; it should be kept in mind that helping to develop practical and applicable thinking as opposed to theoretical or 'dead' knowledge constitutes our prime objective.

These learning materials have been tried and tested in many different countries and with health workers working at different levels. They have been used with professional health workers, particularly with university students or staff in the health services, and also with health personnel at district and local level who have perceived it as a very important incentive to improve their performance.

Diagram 2

The use of different techniques will lend more weight to the results

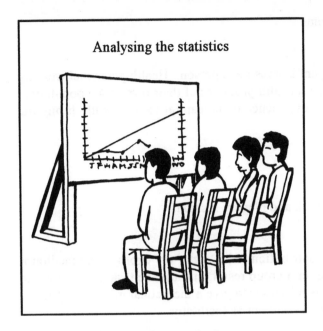

Analysing the statistics

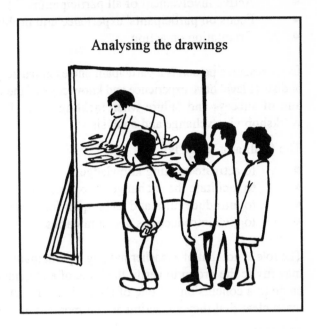

Analysing the drawings

How to Use the Materials

The materials have been designed for two training workshops. Ideally, each should be covered in five days so as to permit the study of additional materials in another 1–2 day training session. Total training could even be spread over a two-week period, or longer. It would be possible to deal with the materials in fewer days, but this would be at the expense of in-depth discussions.

Participants

Participants should be health workers working at district level or in a hospital or health centre and should have some years of professional experience.

Facilitators

The ideal trainee–facilitator ratio should be six to one, a ratio of seven or even eight to one still being acceptable. The total number of facilitators should be not less than five, that of trainees not more than (and preferably less than) 35. An experienced facilitator could supervise and support three different groups simultaneously.

We would like to stress that the health managers involved in the workshop will be expected to put into practice the ideas highlighted during the course, once they step into their supervisory role.

> This book is not only a facilitator's manual, it is also a supervisor's manual

Principles to be applied in the training workshop

Three guiding principles should be applied in the workshop:

- Active involvement of all participants
- Focus on participants' experience and problems
- Orientation on action.

Every resource person is a participant and each participant is a resource person. Health personnel working at district level have experience and knowledge of the main health problems of their own target population, and of success and failure when tackling them. This experience is the capital to work with during the workshop via exchange and analysis.

The facilitator's role is:

- to activate existing knowledge
- to facilitate the exchange of experience
- to introduce rules and techniques for group work and plenary sessions
- to give introductions and summaries.

The role is not that of a teacher judging a participant's contribution to be 'right' or 'wrong'. The facilitator may invite the group to verify the logic of a statement or a group result, but it is the task of the group to come to a conclusion. If one of the facilitators acts as a lecturer to give a theoretical input, it should be made clear that they are acting at that moment as lecturer and not as facilitator.

The interaction between individual work, group work and plenary sessions (and the common visualization of the working process) helps to involve each participant actively in the process.

Focus on participants' experience and problems

The problems discussed in the workshop should be, as far as possible, problems taken from the participants' professional experience and not from theory. The facilitator should try to ensure that the problems analysed are real problems and not drawn from participants' study notes or from literature.

Orientation on action

The overall objective of the district workshop is to develop knowledge, skills and attitudes that can be applied by the health team afterwards. Approaches that are theoretically possible should be evaluated by asking whether they are applicable and under what conditions.

Training methods

During the workshop various training methods will be used:

- short introductions and explanations by the facilitator
- brainstorming sessions based on common sense and scope of experience of the participants
- ordering of drawings
- exercises for group work
- structuring of ideas with the aid of cards and ensuring group discussions
- reading out text
- teaching games
- making graphs.

Diagram 3

Three different methodological approaches

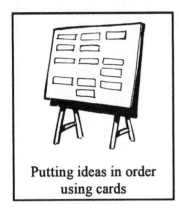

Putting ideas in order using cards

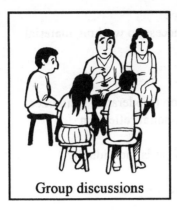

Group discussions

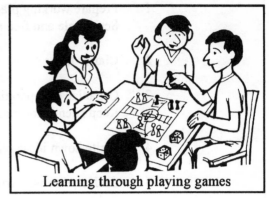

Learning through playing games

Knowing that memory is facilitated by using the eyes in conjunction with listening to lecturers, continuous visualization of ideas and results is suggested. According to the principles mentioned above, this visualization should be generated by all participants.

An interaction between the different methods according to the subject treated and to the group dynamics is the best guarantee of keeping the group actively involved.

In the following paragraph we will provide some details about the educational methods to be used.

Teaching Methods

Working in small groups

In order to increase communication among participants, it is essential to have small groups. Everybody has more of a chance to contribute more often to the discussion. Therefore discussion should take place mainly in the groups. Even if there are not enough rooms to form working groups, small discussion groups could be set up in the same room.

A working group should consist of at least three participants and have not more than seven to allow full participation by everybody.

The application of the following recommendations helps to organize group work efficiently. (They should be prepared on a pinboard or a flip chart and presented to the groups).

Chart 1
Steps in group work

1	Prepare working place Semicircle and free access to working material
2	Clarify tasks
3	Organize co–operation (moderator, visualizor) Keep silence for individual reflection
4	Write down ideas on cards individually
5	Collect, discuss, structure your ideas
6	Fill in anything that is missing
7	Prepare presentation

If a group becomes stuck on a controversial debate and goes round in circles without coming to an agreement, the facilitator should encourage the group to accept the differing points of view, to visualize them and move on. Often the documentation of conflicting ideas enriches the whole discussion. Working in a subgroup does not necessarily mean coming up with a consensus.

Plenary discussion

The presentation of the group work in the plenary session serves to exchange ideas between the different working groups. In order to avoid boring and endless presentations, these should be limited to visualized ideas. What has been discussed but not pinned on the board should not be presented. Often it is useful to set the presentation time in advance, thus avoiding long presentations and guaranteeing equal time for each group.

An important feature of conducting a workshop is the interaction of individual work, small group sessions and plenary sessions. As a rule of thumb it can be said that deep and detailed work belongs to small groups, whereas critical analysis and different forms of idea-collection are better conducted in a large group.

Diagram 4

Suggestions for the presentation of group work

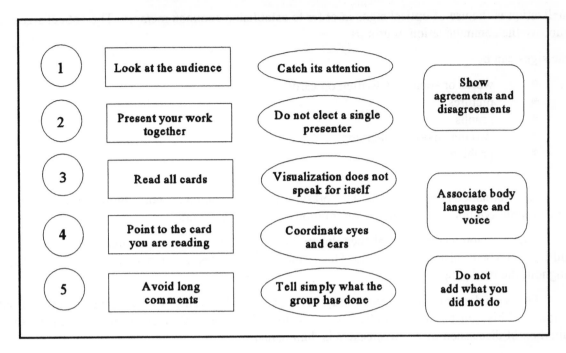

A plenary discussion in a large group of 30 to 40 participants needs some discipline if it is to be fruitful. In order to avoid 'relapse' into pupil–teacher behaviour, the group should agree on the framework and rules of discussion.

Most important are

- a common understanding of the subject of discussion

- an agreement on the time accorded to one session (the election of a time–controller, who reminds participants of the remaining time, is helpful)

- agreement on a discussion leader who gives permission to speak and keeps a watch on the duration of individual contributions and on the sequence of speakers.

The visualization of the main results of a plenary discussion is a rather useful method. It helps in reaching a consensus and avoids repetitions. It ensures that everybody is able to follow and helps to detect misunderstandings early. One of the facilitators should play the role of secretary of the plenary discussion by writing down the main ideas mentioned on cards and pinning them continually on a board. Reading out this 'protocol' at the end of the discussion gives a summary for the whole group and a chance to add any missing ideas.

Mobile visualization

What do we mean by visualization?

Visualization is the use of optical signs in order to establish a common memory. The optical signs serve to improve the communication in groups.

These signs can be

- words or sentences written on cards
- pictures
- graphs
- two dimensional diagrams
- problem trees.

All information provided during the workshop and all participants' contributions are written in big letters, graphic symbols or pictorial representations visible to everyone.

The common memory established during the workshop reduces repetitions, discussions that go round in circles and misunderstandings. The visualization creates a common stock of ideas accessible throughout the workshop.

The visualization allows everybody to write what he wants, to contribute to each problem mentioned. This can be done simultaneously so that the degree of interaction is increased and the domination of discussion by a few speakers is diminished.

What do we mean by mobile visualization? Mobile visualization means that file cards are used for writing. Each idea is written on a separate card instead of being written on a blackboard, a transparency or a flip chart. This method allows the clustering and structuring of ideas and the establishment of relationships (e.g. by using arrows to order ideas in two-dimensional diagrams). It allows the documentation of a participatory group process by rearranging the cards, after ideas and concepts have been developed.

Learning to write legibly presents some difficulties. Adults often regard handwriting as an expression of their personality and not as a communication tool. Another problem is the use of very long sentences or only keywords, instead of writing short sentences. The rules presented in Diagram 5 can help to increase legibility. They should be prepared in advance on a pin board or on a big sheet, presented to the group and respected as far as possible by everybody.

Collecting and structuring ideas

To give each participant the same chance to contribute their ideas on a given question, individual writing on cards is an effective method.

Each group member must have easy access to the visualization material. Everybody should have sufficient time to formulate his or her ideas. The cards should not be pinned to the board until everybody has finished writing.

The number of cards should be limited to a total of 50 or 60 per question in order to allow its management on the pinboard. A limited number of cards per participant is thus agreed.

The facilitator collects the cards, reads out each one slowly and then pins it to the pinboard. All cards are accepted. Even if a statement is not clear, it is read out. The facilitator should invite the group to clarify the meaning, and avoids questions like: 'Who has written this card?' Nobody should be forced to 'confess'. If the author of a card wants to clarify the meaning or to reformulate the card he/she could do so. The facilitator should avoid giving personal judgements on any cards. It is the task of the group to decide whether the meaning is clear.

Arranging the cards on the pinboard can be done

- by clustering, that means forming groups of ideas under one heading (e.g. collection of main health problems)
- by ordering them in a pre-established diagram (e.g. measures to cope with a health problem)
- by ordering them in a cause–effect relationship. (e.g. causation tree)

Diagram 5
Rules and reasons in the use of writing types

You should use the broad edge of a marker pen

Your handwriting may say something about you but at times it can be difficult to read

WRITING VISUALLY

Full recognition from 8 metres away

RULES	REASONS	AVOID
One idea, one card	For better structuring	Too many thoughts expressed and incomplete sentences are difficult to read and understand. It will also be hard to separate your ideas from the cluster
A maximum of 3 or 4 ideas on each card	For legibility	
Narrow script is best	Economizes space	This script is far to thin in comparison to its size
		Broadly spaced is more difficult to read than narrow writing
Start writing at the upper left hand corner	Leaves space to add thoughts	If you don't you may not be able to fit everthing you want to say
Use both capital and lower case letters	For faster reading	CAPITAL LETTERS ALONE ARE MORE DIFFICULT TO READ than lower case letters

9

Diagram 6

Structuring ideas by using cards

Playing teaching games

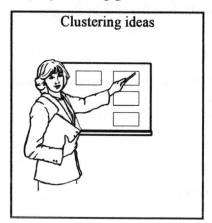
Clustering ideas

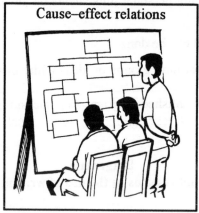
Cause–effect relations

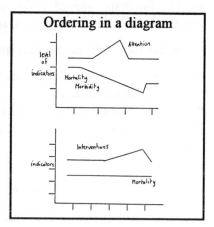
Ordering in a diagram

During the workshop a lot of new information is offered and new terms are introduced. The teaching games in Appendix A.3 and B.3 offer an opportunity to reinforce the acquired knowledge, clarify remaining questions and sum up the main ideas discussed throughout the day.

Instead of closing a module with an evaluation questionnaire, questions are asked in connection with a relaxing activity. The individual has to answer a question and it is the group's task to judge whether an answer is acceptable. The facilitator's role is to clarify questions if needed.   The games chosen are of a familiar pattern and the rules are simple.

To prepare the use of the teaching games the board, the rules and the questions are to be copied according to the number of subgroups. The board is glued on to a piece of pasteboard. The questions are put on to small cards. Dice and pawns sufficient for all groups are prepared.

Organizing a Workshop

The facilitator should have a basic understanding of epidemiology and experience in the management of population-based data. He/she should have read one or more books from those listed.

While preparing a workshop, particular attention should be paid to:

- Budget, sources of financing
- Rooms (there should be one room for each subgroup)
- Materials to be covered
- Timetable
- Invitation to the participants.

Participants should bring with them the following documents (if available):

- annual or monthly reports
- maps of their catchment area
- data about deaths, births, population size and composition
- reports of activities (vaccination, ante-natal care, growth monitoring, etc.).

For materials needed to prepare the workshop, see Chart 2.

Learning Objectives of the Training Course

These training materials are designed for health managers working at district level or at a hospital or health centre to use for on-the-job training of local personnel.

After completion of Part A of this workshop, the health workers should be able to:

1.   enumerate the nine epidemiological questions and apply them in their own work;
2.   define the target population of their health facility;
3.   understand the classification of the population into different age, sex, ethnic and socio–economic groups and use this classification;
4.   identify the high–risk groups in the target communities and adapt existing control strategies to the specific needs of those communities;
5.   know how to monitor the coverage of the target population with health programmes such as vaccination, prenatal care, child development, malaria prophylaxis, etc;
6.   monitor the degree of productivity and efficiency of their health services;
7.   identify an epidemic outbreak.

After completion of Part B, the health workers should be able to:

1.   enumerate the nine epidemiological questions related to health services' problems;
2.   define the main indicators to assess health services and to apply them to the real situation;
3.   elaborate district priorities concerning the health problems and those of the health services;
4.   design an integrated district health plan to improve health status and health services;
5.   monitor and evaluate the different components of a district health plan.

These learning materials do not cover the use of statistical significance tests. They do not deal with the design of epidemiological studies and do not explain the difference between the terms rate and ratio, prevalence and incidence, proportion and rate.

Basic Assumptions for the Success of the Workshop

The following are essential for the successful implementation of epidemiological thinking at local health level:

● supervision of health workers should be continuous and of an acceptable quality
● supervisors must put emphasis on epidemiological thinking and encourage health workers to use it
● sufficient communication and trust must reign between health workers and community on the one hand, and within the health hierarchy on the other
● personnel turnover must be kept low
● collected data must be understood and used by health workers and communities alike. It is the responsibility of supervisors to check not only on the collection of data but also on its use.

Chart 2. Materials to be prepared for the workshop

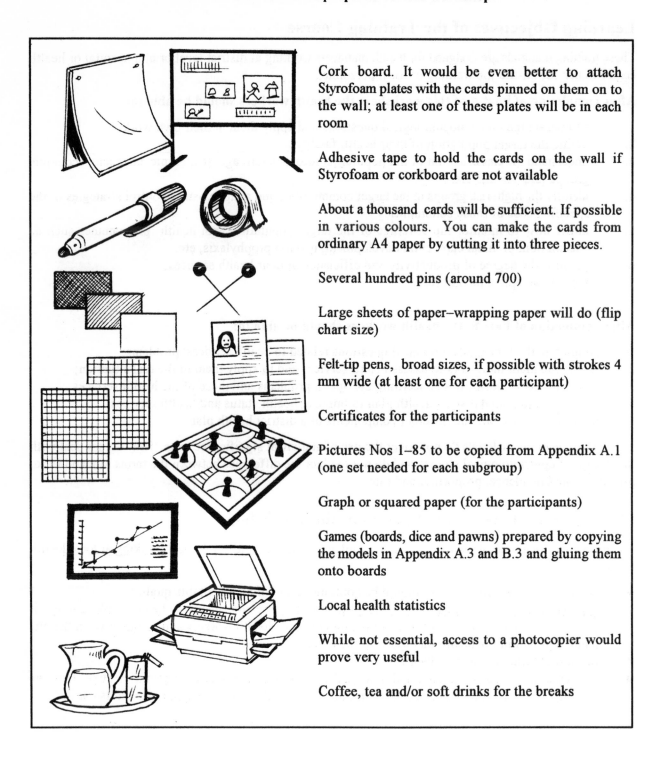

Cork board. It would be even better to attach Styrofoam plates with the cards pinned on them on to the wall; at least one of these plates will be in each room

Adhesive tape to hold the cards on the wall if Styrofoam or corkboard are not available

About a thousand cards will be sufficient. If possible in various colours. You can make the cards from ordinary A4 paper by cutting it into three pieces.

Several hundred pins (around 700)

Large sheets of paper–wrapping paper will do (flip chart size)

Felt-tip pens, broad sizes, if possible with strokes 4 mm wide (at least one for each participant)

Certificates for the participants

Pictures Nos 1–85 to be copied from Appendix A.1 (one set needed for each subgroup)

Graph or squared paper (for the participants)

Games (boards, dice and pawns) prepared by copying the models in Appendix A.3 and B.3 and gluing them onto boards

Local health statistics

While not essential, access to a photocopier would prove very useful

Coffee, tea and/or soft drinks for the breaks

PART A

PART A

WORKSHOP ON THE USE OF EPIDEMIOLOGY AT DISTRICT AND LOCAL LEVEL

Schedule

Four introductory sessions of one-and-a-half to two hours each are to be held every day, two in the morning, two in the afternoon with an occasional additional session in the evening. Each session is followed by a break. The topics to be covered and the tasks to be performed during the course of each session have been determined in advance. It is important, however, to remain flexible and to adapt the progress of the workshop to the specific requirements of a given group of participants. If long discussions arise on one topic, it may prove necessary to halt an unfinished session and to hold an additional one in the evening.

A rough description of the topics to be covered on any given day may look like this:

THE FIVE-DAY WORKSHOP

Day No.	0	1	2	3	4	5
MORNING (2 sessions)	Arrival	Module A1 The nine epidemiological questions (Q.1–Q.9)	Module A2 (cont'd) (Q.2, Q.3)	Module A2 (cont'd) (Q.6)	Module A2 (cont'd) (Q.9)	Module A3 Training in epidemiological thinking
AFTERNOON (2 sessions)	Arrival of facilitators and participants Participants introduce themselves Introduction into the ideas of the workshop	Module A2 Exercises on epidemiological tools (Q.1–Q.4)	Module A2 (cont'd) (Q.4, Q.5)	Module A2 (cont'd) (Q.7, Q.8)	Poster preparation	Final test and evaluation of the workshop

Additional five-hour modules

Module A4
> Who is affected? Risk approach

Module A5
> Model of disease causation and control measures.

Module A6
> An epidemic outbreak.

While an introductory session is held on Sunday afternoon, the workshop itself begins on Monday morning with the first session of instruction.

Structure of the Workshop

QUESTIONS	OBJECTIVES	PROCEDURE	MATERIALS	TIME
MODULE A1				
The nine epidemiological questions. (Q.1–Q.9)	To know the nine epidemiological questions	Presentation by the facilitator Group discussion (brainstorming) First didactic game	Chart with the nine questions Set of questions	2 sessions
MODULE A2				
Q.1 Identification and priority setting of health problems	To produce a list of health problems in the participants specific areas To prioritize the listed health problems	Brainstorming (in groups) Facilitator introduces priority setting. Participants prioritize on the matrix	Cards Priority matrix Felt pens	1 session
Q.2 How many cases occur?	To know possible sources of information To understand the concept of proportion To use pie charts and pictograms	To arrange pictures in rows (in groups) To answer the questions written on cards (groups) Clarify doubts (in groups or plenary sessions) Second didactic game	Pictures (10–17) Cards, corkboard, pictures 18 & 19	2 sessions
Q.3 When do the problems occur?	To know how health problems vary with time	Work with a matrix and pictures Group exercise	Matrix, pictures (21–28) Squared paper	1 session
Q.4 Where do the cases occur?	To learn how to draw a map To know how to use a sketch map	Preparation and interpretation of different sketch maps (in groups)	Corkboard, felt-tip pens	½ session
Q.5 How is the population affected?	To know about risk groups and risk factors	Identify associations between certain diseases and population groups/characteristics through pictures	Pictures (29–52) Cards, pens, board with definitions	1 ½ sessions

QUESTIONS	OBJECTIVES	PROCEDURE	MATERIALS	TIME
Q.6 Why does the problem occur?	Analyse the cause–effect relationship in a diagram (problem tree)	Facilitator introduces concept Elaboration of the problem tree (in groups) Comparison among trees produced	Corkboard, cards, pens	2 sessions
Q.7 and Q.8 What kind of measures have been taken? What results or difficulties have been found?	To classify prevention of primary, secondary or tertiary care. To classify measures taken	Exercise using pictures Exercise using the intervention matrix	Pictures (54–56) Matrix, corkboard	2 sessions
Q.9 What else could be done?	Learning to do the objective tree and the planning matrix	Introduction by facilitator Objective tree (in groups) Use of the matrix	Corkboard, cards, pens Matrix	2 sessions
Poster preparation	To know how to present condensed information by using a poster	Introduction by facilitator Preparation of the poster Marking of posters and discussion	Corkboard, cards, pens, scissors	4 sessions
MODULE A3				
Training in epidemiological thinking	Analyse an epidemic outbreak	Read a text To carry out the tasks (in groups)	Copies of the exercise Paper	1 or 2 sessions

MODULE A1. THE NINE EPIDEMIOLOGICAL QUESTIONS

Plenary session

1. Pin a large piece of paper (1.5 m by 2 m, or larger), with the nine epidemiological questions clearly printed, on the Styrofoam plates or corkboard fastened on the wall.

THE NINE EPIDEMIOLOGICAL QUESTIONS

A.	**IDENTIFICATION**	
	Q.1	What are the main health problems in your community or district?
B.	**MAGNITUDE AND DISTRIBUTION**	
	Q.2	How many cases or health events did you come across?
	Q.3	When do these generally occur? (a particular time of the year, a particular week, a specific day?)
	Q.4	Where do they occur? (Are they limited to a particular area? Indicate location on the map)
	Q.5	Who is affected? (particular individuals, men more than women or vice versa, the very young, the young, the old, families, ethnic groups? Are people of the same income level, with similar occupations, habits, or family structure more affected than others?)
C.	**ANALYSIS**	
	Q.6	Why does the problem occur? (What are the main factors involved here?)
D.	**MEASURES TAKEN**	
	Q.7	What kind of measures did you yourself and/or others take to deal with the problem?
	Q.8	What results did you achieve? What difficulties did you encounter in trying to deal with the problem?
	Q.9	What else could be done? What kind of assistance is needed?

Note: Use markers of different colours to write the phrases and/or sentences inside the parentheses.

2. Read the questions aloud and explain that they will form the core of the entire workshop.
3. Define, together with the participants, the word 'epidemiology'. At the end of this exercise, you can pin on the board the following:

> EPIDEMIOLOGY is the study of the distribution and determinants of health problems and disease in human populations. The purpose of epidemiology is to obtain, interpret and use health information to promote health and reduce disease.

(Vaughan and Morrow 1989)

Q.1	What are the main health problems in your community or district?

1. Ask the participants the following question: 'What are the main health problems in your community?' This pertains only to health events (diseases, low weight, disabilities, etc.), *not to health service-related problems.*

Each participant then lists one to three problems on one to three different cards, which are gathered and pinned on the Styrofoam-covered wall or corkboard.

2. The facilitator reads out the cards after collecting them and forms clusters of the same or similar ideas (see: notes on Teaching Methods, p. 5).
3. Divide the participants into small groups of six to eight persons. Each group gets a list of the nine epidemiological questions. Before splitting up, each group selects one of the major health problems (a different one for each group) already identified and to be discussed. The problem must be clearly defined in order to avoid misunderstandings.
4. Group work: each group now has answers to the health problem they have selected within the framework of Questions 2 to 9.
5. Each group should write on the cards or on paper its own conclusions in the form of keywords or very short phrases.
6. Presentation of results in a plenary session.

Ideally, there should be one facilitator per group. However, since this is not always possible, one facilitator can cover two or three groups at a time. The facilitator's main responsibility is to stimulate and structure discussion within the various groups while *joining in as little as possible him/herself.*

Facilitator's guide for supporting the brainstorming on the epidemiological questions

---

Q.2	How many cases or health events did you come across?

Ask each group to discuss its answer to the health problem it has selected and to come to a conclusion on 'how big' that problem actually is in its own district or province, or catchment area. The answer should derive entirely from the experience and knowledge of the group members or from the information they are handling or producing.

Ask each group to write a very detailed answer on a piece of paper or, better still, on a card that can then be shown to the other groups.

In formulating their answers, the group may come upon new questions which must also be answered when determining how big a health problem actually is. Some of the issues which might come up are:

- How do we count the cases or health events occurring in our area? What units do we use? (e.g. consultations, deaths, illness in the community).

- What sources of information do we have for answering this question? (e.g. epidemiological surveillance and other reports; patients' cards or files; attaching colour tags to the cards of patients at risk–an easy way to readily identify problem cases in the unit's archive).

- How does the number of events relate to the size of the population in which they occur? (Here you have a basis from which we can introduce the concept of rate).

If, when listening to the discussions, you notice that group members are raising these or similar issues, comment on it and get them to incorporate these issues in their group answer to Question 2. But do this only if the groups raise these issues themselves (in a spontaneous way). Do not bring it up yourself and do not give any explanations at this stage. That will come later (Module A2).

Q.3	When do the cases or health events generally occur?

Proceed as for Question 2, asking each group to write a detailed answer to the questions, derived from its own experience and knowledge.

As you did previously, encourage the groups to record any useful ideas for secondary questions, but do not forget that you may do this only after the ideas or secondary questions have cropped up in the discussion, unprompted. For example:

- How can 'when' be defined? In terms of dates and/or time periods? (years, months, weeks, days) in terms of useful milestones? (festivities, fairs.)
- What sources of information do we have to answer this question? (records, fairs.)
- How can time changes be presented? This could form the basis for a discussion of time charts, or time series.
- What aspects of case evolution have surfaced in the discussion? This could prove useful for introducing the notions of long-term trends, cyclic variations, outbreaks.

Q.4	Where do the cases or health events occur?

Proceed as for Questions 2 and 3.

In this case (discussion of spatial distribution of cases or events), watch for spontaneous secondary questions concerning:

- sources of information
- usefulness of presenting the answer with the help of a map or a sketch of the area.

As before, make a brief comment about it and suggest that the group include these ideas in its answer.

Q.5	Who is affected by the cases or health events?

Proceed as above. In their answers, the group should describe (in the form of a list) individuals who do or do not suffer from cases of ill-health and those who are or are not affected by health events.

If, and only if, the group presents a spontaneous classification of the characteristics of persons, families or villages associated with the problem, you should remark that 'it might be a good thing' to include this in the answer as well.

Q.6   Why does the problem occur?

Proceed as above.

The groups' answers should be in the form of lists of possible causes and factors. Emphasize once again that all this should come from their local experience. Warn them (with a smile) that they may have been told or taught about 'the causes of problem x' and that what they have learned may not necessarily be true for their area. They are about to create their own knowledge and come to their own conclusions. The possible causes should be determined by the groups on the basis of their previous answers to:

- When do the cases or health events generally occur?
- Where do they occur?
- Who is affected?

Suggest that before listing each cause, they also indicate the reasons why they have done so. Primarily they should seek these reasons in their answers to the three previous questions, but they may also look for them elsewhere.

If, and only if, the groups begin to think in terms of a) classification of causes, and b) a possible relationship between these causes, should you encourage them to include this in their answers.

Q.7   What kind of measures did you yourself and others in the community take to cope with the problem?

The basic answer of the groups is expected to emerge in the form of a list of interventions (solutions) that they deem appropriate for alleviating the problem.

Suggest that before they list the interventions, they indicate first which cause(s) a given intervention is supposed to deal with. Also ask them to write down any relationships they may perceive between the interventions.

The groups should also mention the kind of interventions that were considered and then abandoned, indicate which new ones are currently being implemented and whether any are in the planning stage.

This will give the group a clearer picture of what has been tried, what is currently being implemented and what may be considered.

Q.8   What results have been achieved? What kinds of difficulties did you encounter in trying to deal with the problem?

The answers of the groups will probably be a description of changes that the participants attribute to their interventions. These changes may be of several kinds–in health, in health care, in government and community opinions, etc. The groups should be encouraged to focus on the changes in health status of their respective communities.

Before describing the changes, they should indicate which interventions they think brought them about.

Since most participants probably encountered difficulties in their attempts to carry out the interventions or in achieving results, these difficulties should be listed. While doing this, some groups may spontaneously elect to use greater precision when reporting on the quantity, quality and distribution of the interventions or related activities. The facilitator should encourage this.

Q.9	What else could be done? What kind of assistance is needed?

The groups should now be instructed to examine again the difficulties and obstacles they encountered while tackling the health problems. In front of each difficulty or obstacle listed, they should indicate whatever means they think might help to overcome it.

Some of these means may lie outside the realm of the local health system; they may be available only at some higher level of the health sector or in some other services; they may become available only after the relevant legislation has been passed, or depend on membership in voluntary associations, etc.

The groups may report on whether they think the additional means that are available might be applied at all, and if so, on how they would work to advantage.

At the end of the plenary session in the morning, you can play the first didactic game. This game is called 'The Snail' and it lasts approximately 40 minutes. (Appendix A.3).

MODULE A2. EXERCISES WITH EPIDEMIOLOGICAL TOOLS

Panel exercise

Q.1	What are the main common health problems in your community?

Go back to the list of health problems identified.

Introduce the need for *setting priorities!*

Various methods can be used for setting priorities. They are based on economic considerations, demands of health care and others. A more comprehensive way of setting priorities is shown below.

Display the following table on a wall chart:

List of health problems	Frequency 'How often'	Severity[1] 'How severe?'	People's concern [2] 'Are people worried?	Sensitivity to public health measures[3] 'Can something useful be done?'	TOTAL
1.					
2.					
3.					
etc.					

1. Severity: in terms of numbers of deaths from the disease and in terms of people disabled as a result of the disease.

2. People's concern: in terms of social stigma attached to the disease (those stricken are rejected by the community) and in terms of fear.

3. Sensitivity to public health measures: (a) in terms of the feasibility of control (can anything be done?) and; (b) in terms of costs (is it cheap or expensive to control the problem?).

Each participant has the right to enter up to ten points in each column. These points are 'votes' which the participant draws (or applies to sticky areas on the paper, provided that these have been reserved for that purpose) next to the health problems that the participant thinks are most frequent, severe, etc. After all participants have cast their votes, these are added so as to assign each health problem a place in the list (order of occurrence or of priority). The group then discusses whether this order matches its expectations and experiences.

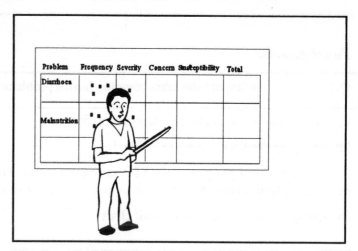

| Q.2 | How many cases or health events did you come across? |

Group exercise

1. In all rooms where group work is to take place, a wall sheet or, better still, a corkboard or a Styrofoam board with the drawings must be at hand.
2. Once this is done, the participants should discuss how they would themselves proceed in their respective settings in order to get the necessary information.

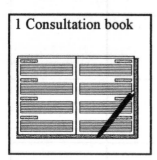
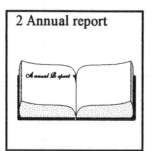
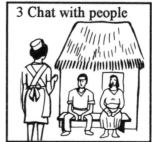
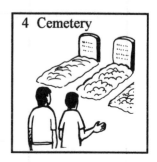

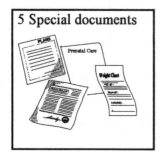
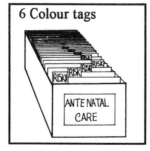
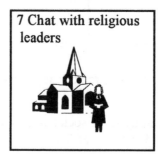
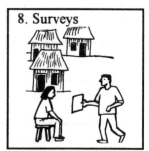

Proportions and graphical representation

Group exercise

1.   Look at the following drawings:

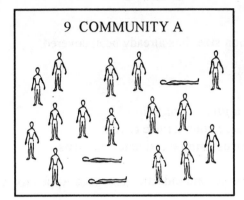 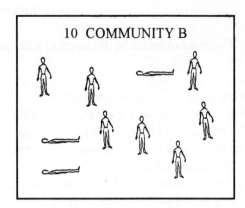

In these two communities you can see healthy people standing, and sick people lying down.

2.   Answer the following questions (the facilitators have the questions on cards which will be given out to the participants):

   (a)   Which community is healthier and why?

   (b)   What is meant by the *proportion* of sick and disabled people in a given community? Determine the proportion of sick people in Communities A and B.

   (c)   Can you represent the proportions you have just calculated as segments of a pie chart?

   (d)   Can you draw the same proportions in the form of a row of people, some of them healthy, the rest sick? (This is called a *pictogram*).

3.   The participants now have to calculate proportions from real data provided by the facilitators and present it graphically in the form of pie charts and pictograms.

4.   If time permits, explain 'Infant Mortality Rate' and 'Maternal Mortality Rate.' They are useful indicators of the health status of a given population.

$$\text{Infant mortality rate} = \frac{\text{No. of deaths among children less than 1 year old in one year}}{\text{No. of live births in the same year}} \times 1{,}000$$

$$\text{Maternal mortality rate} = \frac{\text{No. of maternal deaths}^{1}\text{ in a given area in one year}}{\text{No. of live births in the same area in the same year.}} \times 1,000$$

5.   'The need to relate health events to the population size' has already been covered.

Discuss:
(a)   What does *population size* mean?
(b)   Where and how do we obtain data on the *size of a given population* ?
No. of households in the catchment area (i.e. the area your service covers)
No. of persons in the catchment area, national census, annual estimates, tax lists, microcensus, others.
Should 30–45 minutes remain available, you can play the second didactic game (see Appendix A.3). Otherwise, you can play it in the evening.

SECOND DAY OF THE WORKSHOP

Q.3	When do the cases or events generally occur?

Group exercise

1.   Variation of the health problems over time

Pictures of the following events and conditions ('health events') are displayed on the wall (on a wall sheet, flip chart or flannelograph) for the group to see.

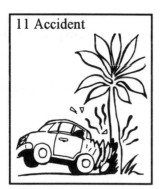
11 Accident

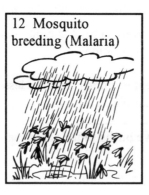
12 Mosquito breeding (Malaria)

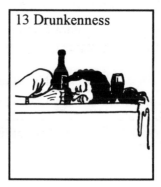
13 Drunkenness

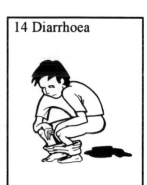
14 Diarrhoea

---

[1] 'Maternal deaths' means deaths related to pregnancy, childbirth and puerperal period.

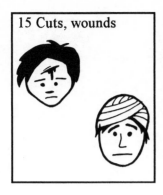

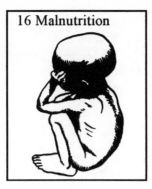

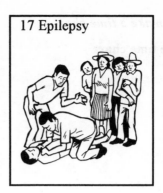

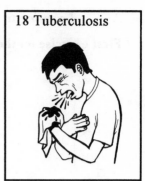

Arrange them in different rows as shown below. Discuss the options.

Many health problems *vary according to:*	Health problems	Comments
the time of the year (seasonal variation)		
the time of the week		
the time of the day		
show no marked variation		

Provide other examples of health events occurring in your area at any particular time. (Write them on cards and pin them up.)

You can also mention the implications for the health services (see Module B1, page 53).

2.   *Learning to make a time chart*

First exercise on the time chart

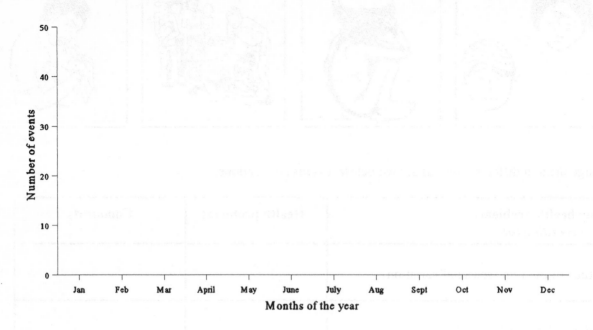

The facilitator explains the graphical presentation of health events occurring during the course of a year. (Each participant is given graph or squared paper and asked to draw the horizontal and vertical line as shown above.)

The following annual report of a given health centre shows for every month of the year the number of patients (children) attending the health centre. Does it reflect the actual situation in your area?

Month	Number of patients	Month	Number of patients
January	5	July	8
February	12	August	6
March	40	September	5
April	35	October	4
May	26	November	6
June	14	December	5

(a) The participants draw a linear graph.
(b) They discuss and try to explain the shape of the graph.
(c) They are asked to take other examples from their area. These examples should be based on documents and reports from their own health centre, and show seasonal variations. They should now practice making linear graphs.

Second exercise on the time chart

(a) Draw a vertical line and a horizontal one
(b) Draw a diagram using the following data

Month	Number of patients admitted to hospital	
	Due to diarrhoea	Due to cholera
January	10	4
February	15	3
March	70	1
April	65	2
May	62	4
June	64	8
July	68	6
August	102	15
September	145	61
October	106	20
November	98	22
December	50	12

(c) Draw a linear graph and put a title to it
(d) Discuss the possible implications of seasonal variations to this data
(e) What could you do to minimize these variations? Use examples taken from the participants' experiences.

Q.4	Where do the cases or health events occur?

Group exercise

1. *Learning to draw a map* **(A simple map or sketch)**

(a) Read the following instructions on the wall:

> List the features you think should be included on a map representing your work area.
> How would you draw these features?

After the participants have finished drawing their list of features (roads, pathways, houses or villages, rivers, health posts, etc.), discuss with them how to draw these items on the map.

(b) They should now draw a map of the catchment area of their own health facility.

(c) Distances from these catchment areas to their respective facilities (expressed in kilometres and/or travel time) as well as the population size of their own communities are to be drawn using different colours.

(d) Particular places/communities where particular health events (diseases, malnutrition, etc.) occur are to be marked with pins.

(e)   For comparison purposes, display in the main room the participants' various sketches. (Should you wish to do so, you can also award prizes to the authors of the best ones).

2.   *Multiple use of simplified maps*

The chief medical director of a health centre carried out a census in the five communities (which have no interconnection) within its catchment area. The data collected is as follows:

Community	Number of inhabitants	Distance to the Health Centre
A	2023	15 minutes
B	501	60 minutes
C	356	2 hours
D	722	2 hours
E	818	4 hours

(a)   Make a map or sketch using this data

(b)   To what ends could this map be used?

(c)   What else could/should be included in the sketch?

(d)   Draw a sketch of your own work area which should portray:

   •   the health posts (or health units) and their distances from the main health centre
   •   the necessary information for a vaccination campaign and supervisory visits.

Q5.   Who is affected?

Group exercise

1.   *Identifying population characteristics and how to classify them*

The group now can look at various pictures (copied from Appendix 1) displayed on the wall sheet, or corkboard. They show several population characteristics and groups of people to be found in a given community.

(a)   Ask the group to write down on cards other population characteristics and to add these to the pictures.

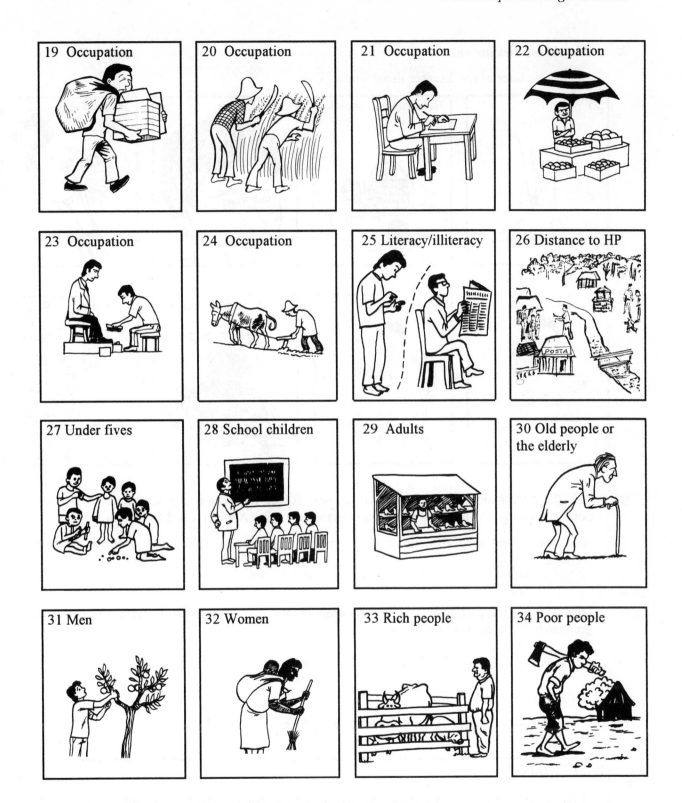

(b)   Discuss possible associations between these characteristics and put the relevant cards together.

2. *Identifying risk groups*

Display pictures of the diseases listed below.

35 Wound	36 Burns and scalds	37 Measles	38 Back pain
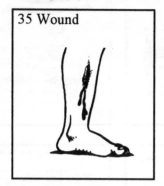	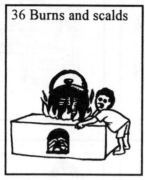	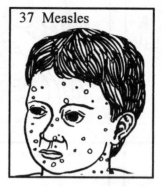	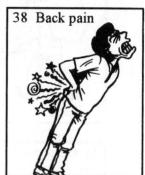

39 Malnutrition	40 Alcoholism	41 Birth problems	42 Obesity
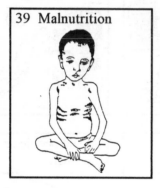	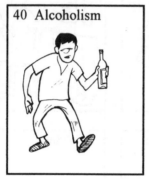	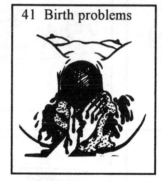	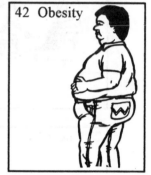

(a) Ask the participants to pin these pictures next to the population characteristics or groups of population with which they are frequently associated. (See Appendix A.2 for solutions).

Additionally, ask them to write on cards any other damages to health and pin them beside the pictures.

(b) Discuss with the participants why these associations between certain diseases and population groups/characteristics actually exist.

(c) Introduce the concepts of *risk factor* and *risk group*.

3. *Definition of 'risk'*

(a) Pin the following charts on the wall and discuss the concept of risk

---
RISK FACTOR

A risk factor can be defined as a variable that entails the increased probability of contracting a given disease through exposure and/or susceptibility to it.

(Vaughan & Morrow 1989)

> **RISK GROUP**
>
> A risk group is a group of people who are (or have been) exposed to risk factors and are therefore at a greater risk of contracting a given disease.

(b) Find additional examples of risk factors, write each one on a different piece of paper and pin them on the wall (see also Module 4).

(c) Group the risks from the previous exercise into risks by occupation, age, sex, etc.

(d) Discuss the following point with the participants:

How can we identify risk groups in our catchement area? Write the question onto cards and hand them out to the groups (Appendix A2.)

The exercise could be extended to risk factors and risk groups using the material from Module A4.

THIRD DAY OF THE WORKSHOP

Q.6	Why does the problem occur?

Group exercise

1. *Making a 'causation tree.'*

By this, we mean the graphic representation of a hypothetical model of causes and effects explaining the rate of occurrence of a particular disease or health problem (see 'facilitator's guide', page 34).

After lunch, the group is given a set of health statistics of the area where the workshop is held. These statistics are to serve as a basis for the next question.

2. *Quantifying the problems*

1. Try to quantify all problems shown in the 'tree' using the data from your own area. You may have data on:

    - leading causes of death
    - leading diseases or disabilities as diagnosed in your hospital's outpatient clinic
    - activities (last year's) of each team of staff
    - coverage (vaccinations, prenatal care, growth monitoring, etc.).

2. Write this data on the relevant cards of your causation tree.

3. If you are unable to find actual data for some items, write down other possible sources of information (e.g. surveys, group interviews, documents from ministries).

Later, in the afternoon session, the groups will compare their causation trees and discuss the different solutions they have come up with.

During the last 45 minutes of the afternoon session, they will play the third didactic game in groups (see Appendix A3), with questions on maps, catchment areas, risk approach, coverage, etc.

3.   *Facilitator's Guide*

Making the causation tree (example to be found in Appendix A.4).

1. Use a corkboard or wall-chart, and hand out a fair amount of paper (or large cards) and pins.

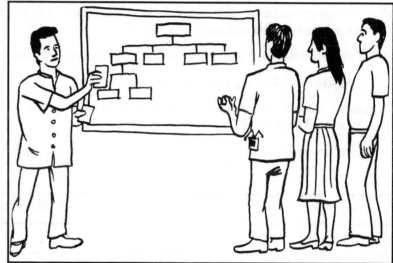

2. Name the key problem the group wants to analyse (it may be the same as on the first day), write it on a card and pin it on the board. It is useful for this exercise that such a key problem reflects a negative event or condition.

3. Ask the participants to write as many causes of the problem they can think of on pieces of paper or cards. Write one idea on one card. At least at the beginning, it might prove useful for each participant to write no more than two or three cards.

4. Collect the cards and read them aloud before pinning them to the corkboard.

5. Ask the group to help arrange the cards on the corkboard in a logical way, in a causation tree. If there are too many cards in any one group, it often proves useful to split into two or more subgroups.

6. Choose a title for each group of ideas on the board.

7. At this point, you and the participants should check whether their ideas (causes of the key health problem under analysis) have been grouped in a logical manner, i.e. whether a 'because of relationship' is always apparent between cause and problem. If this is not the case, the group may decide to remove the irrelevant ideas from the analysis, or reorganize the layout (e.g. to order ideas as sub-causes of causes).

8. Along with the group, you are now to decide whether all possible causes of the problem have been named. Here, new cards for causes and subcauses can be added. They can be written by both the facilitator and the participants.

9. You will now have a causation tree. (You may now reproduce the tree on a sheet of paper, photocopy it and distribute it to the participants. An example of a rather detailed causation tree can be found in Appendix A.4.)

FOURTH DAY OF THE WORKSHOP

Q.7	What kind of measures did you yourself or others in the community take to cope with the problem?

Q.8	What results have been achieved? What kind of difficulties did you encounter in trying to deal with the problem?

Group exercise

Point out that these two questions are related to the diagnosis of the actual situation though they do not refer to damages to health, but to measures taken. These aspects will be dealt with in Part B of this book.

1. Type of intervention

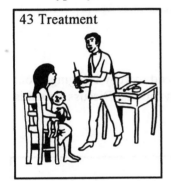
43 Treatment

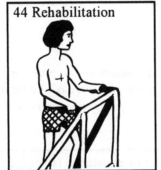
44 Rehabilitation

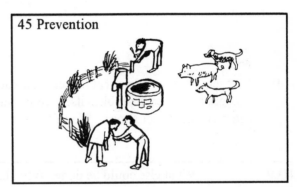
45 Prevention

(a) Show the three drawings that deal with health interventions. How do they differ from the interventions you carry out in your area? How would you label each of them?

(b) Talk about *Prevention*, *Treatment* and *Rehabilitation* (you can introduce the terms primary, secondary, tertiary prevention).

2. Measures taken: difficulties and results.

Now, go back to the causation tree.

(a) Mark with a number those cards which already represent the kind of intervention actually performed by participants.

(b) Write on cards (bearing corresponding numbers) the name of the respective intervention, on others the difficulties encountered, and on a third set the results achieved.

(c) Mark the changes on the cards with +++ or ++ or +, or with *N* or *NN* or *NNN*. If possible, express the changes in numbers.

<table>
<tr><td colspan="6">WHAT KIND OF MEASURES (INTERVENTIONS) DID YOU TAKE TO DEAL WITH THE PROBLEM?</td></tr>
</table>

Number of causes or problems	Which?	How much? (quantity)	How well done? (quality)	Results Changes*
◯				
◯				
◯				

<u>Intervention</u>

(d) You should now explain that reducing the causal factors of the problem, and thereby bringing about changes in the health problem itself, constitutes the *objective* of the interventions. Discuss how this can be measured or shown. We call this measurable objective *target*.

Q.9	What else could be done? What kind of assistance is needed?

Group work

A   *Making a tree of objectives out of the causation tree*

(See Appendix A.4 for an example of tree of objectives.)*

We will now draw the participants' attention back to the 'causation tree' they were asked to 'build' in the previous session. In fact, by beginning with a problem, seeking out and finding its causes and related subcauses, i.e. its 'roots', we ended with an inverted 'tree'. The logical sequence of the argument allowed us to establish 'because of' relationships between causes and subcauses. If we now want to resolve the problem we identified we will have to set ourselves objectives that will have to be achieved. The logical sequence of our causation tree enables us, by simple rewording, to establish objectives and sub-objectives that, in turn, will have to be achieved in order to solve the stated problem.

---

* For the sake of brevity and simplicity, it is possible to skip part A of this exercise and start at part B. Here, you can first incorporate some important problems (or some of the main difficulties identified in the previous session) into the causation tree.

Problems were described as negative states (e.g., insufficiency of..., lack of..., poor ...). By re–phrasing the problems as positive conditions, they take on the form of objectives (... improved, ... replaced, ... on schedule).

1. Reattach the causation tree to the wall for everyone to see. Then begin with rewording the cards on the tree as positive conditions. To this end, use new cards and a pen of a different colour, but retain the same structure.

2. Should you run into difficulties with the rewording, work out what you were really trying to say when stating the problem and seek group agreement.

3. Avoid systematic converse rewording without first considering the sense of the target phrase (e.g., the problem 'increasing demand for curative care' does not necessarily entail the objective 'decreasing demand for curative care'; 'unstable soil' must not become 'stable soil', etc.)

4. Make sure that the cause–effect relationship of the problem analysis is converted into means–end relationships ('sub-objective X in order to achieve sub-objective Y'). But note that not every cause–effect relationship automatically becomes a means–end relationship (e.g. 'loss of traditional feeding habits' as a cause of malnutrition cannot be converted into 'existence of traditional feeding habits' but into 'promotion of adequate feeding habits').

5. The resulting tree of objectives enables us to look at several alternatives (or approaches) that will in turn enable us to reach our final objective. Selecting one or more of these approaches will thus merely be contingent on the available funds, cost-benefit considerations, as well as on their technical and socio-political feasibility.

B   The matrix of activities

1. In the tree of objectives, assign a number to those cards on which the participants indicated that they wanted to launch activities or initiate interventions.

2. Transfer the numbers onto the wall chart and, next to each objective, write down the respective activity/intervention, the target (using an indicator whenever possible) and the basic assumptions/conditions which you consider necessary to reach the target.

No.	Activity	Objective*	Target*	Assumptions/conditions
1				
2				
3				
4				

* Objective: not necessarily measurable; Target: a measurable entity.

During the Plenary Session you will compare group results and discuss the following:

●   are the results realistic?
●   how much time will it take to reach the target?
●   which indicators can be used to measure progress?
●   have the basic assumptions/conditions been correctly stated, has anything been left out?

Designing a poster on the health problems in our area of work

After you have worked on the nine epidemiological questions, you may apply the knowledge acquired in a practical way to the local situation of each participant.

If the participants have the necessary data, you can do the following exercise during the afternoon session on day four, and, if necessary, you can work on it in the following morning's session. Or you can give this exercise as homework.

Main tasks of the exercise:
(a)   Produce a document with the diagnosis of health and health services of your area.
(b)   Present the local health situation in the form of a poster, in a simplified way.
(c)   In a sketch, present the main data relating to health and health-service problems in the area.
        (If there is only enough time for one task then do task b).

Instructions for poster preparation

Approximate size: 2.0 m x 1.5 m.

Information:

- Title (summarizes the contents)
- Geographic, demographic, socio-economic and cultural characteristics as long as they are necessary to understand the following points.
- Description and analysis of the health situation by means of indicators and/or short statements.
- Description and analysis of the health services as above.
- Programmes and activities in progress, including objectives and priority setting.

The Poster must have the following characteristics:

- Be attractive and clear in its presentation
- Data must correspond to reality
- Apply the risk approach
- Have logic coherence taking into account the points mentioned under the title 'information'.

Avoid:

- Excess information
- The absence of a conceptual framework (hypothetical model)
- Proposed actions that are not in line with the rest of the information
- A lack of logical flow within arguments
- A title that does not summarize the poster message.

The poster will be marked by tutors and participants (excluding one's own poster) as very good, good or deficient, taking into account the following criteria:

- Clarity of arrangement
- Attractiveness of presentation
- Logic and rationale underlying the presentation
- Use of risk approach or of indicators.

The tutor and participants mark the poster using the following table. They also write their comments on cards and put them by the poster.

Table for marking the poster

3 = Very good
2 = Good
1 = Deficient

Poster N°	Attractiveness	Clarity and Logic Flow	Use of Risk Approach	Use of Indicators	Total
1					
2					
3					
4					
5					
6					

FIFTH DAY OF THE WORKSHOP

MODULE A3. TRAINING IN EPIDEMIOLOGICAL THINKING

On the last day of the workshop, each group discusses a case study. The nine epidemiological questions are applied to the following story.

Measles in your district

Baseline information

Your workplace is a district health centre. The district stretches over 100 kilometres from the north to the south and some 50 kilometres from the east to the west, and has a total population of about 52,000 (Table 1). According to demographic estimates, 45% of the population in your district is below the age of 15, infant mortality rate is 146 per thousand, under-fives mortality is 243 per thousand and maternal mortality is 6.8 per thousand live births (hospital data only).

The district health services comprise a district health centre with five communal dispensaries, one of which is operated by a missionary group. Apart from a large number of traditional healers (who are not organized into a group), and some health-centre nurses holding private evening clinics, no private medical care is available. Drugs are sold in a central district pharmacy run by a government agency but outside the district medical officer's jurisdiction. The district health centre employs about 15 health workers. Each of the dispensaries is staffed by a nurse and two auxiliaries (see Table 2 for staff distribution and formal qualifications).

Preventive services are essentially restricted to immunization campaigns. These are conducted by mobile government teams at a provincial level. Integrated preventive and curative services can be offered only at health-centre level as this is the only service to possess a refrigerator. Although environmental health surveillance teams do not exist, screening for high-risk patients (children under five years of age and pregnant women) has recently been introduced in the form of clinics held in the district health centre and the communal dispensaries. Small-scale farming constitutes the essential means of subsistence and is the only source of income for the district population, the small cotton crop and part of the food crops being sold to private traders.

Map of the district

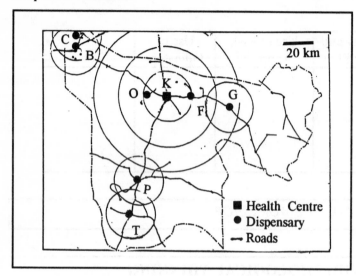

Table 1. Population of the District

Sub district	No. of villages	Total Population
K	11	653
O	10	6,911
F	7	4,442
G	10	6,101
B	7	4,592
C	6	3,422
P	16	16,036
T	7	4,940
Total	74	47,097

Table 2. Staff distribution and qualification

Health Unit	Qualification/staff category	Number
Dispensary B	Enrolled Nurse	1
	Auxiliary	1
Dispensary C (private)	Midwife	2
	Registered Nurse	2
	Auxiliary	6
Dispensary G	Enrolled Nurse	1
	Auxiliary	1
	Auxiliary Midwife	1
Dispensary P	Registered Nurse	1
	Enrolled Nurse	1
	Auxiliary	1
Dispensary T	Enrolled Nurse	2
	Auxiliary	1
Health Centre	Medical Doctor	2
	Midwife	1
	Registered Nurse	2
	Enrolled Nurse	4
	Auxiliary Midwife	4
	Auxiliary	4
	Driver	1

The problem

On 26 March, you receive a written message from the nurse of the northern dispensary in G, informing you that a few cases of measles have been reported by village F (45 families, total population of 275), located on the northern border of the district. The nurse informs you that the villagers strongly suspect witchcraft may be at play, as there have been no cases of measles in the village for at least six years. The villagers do not seek help at the dispensary (which is difficult to reach because of a mountain range and bad roads) and have not seen a mobile medical team for a number of years. An agricultural extension worker who visited the village in the previous week confirms the measles outbreak and informs you that the village chief/headman has imposed a quarantine on every family struck down by the disease: women and their children are required to stay in shelters located in men's fields and are not allowed to visit the family compound in the village. It turns out that measles cases have occurred in about two-thirds of the families. Children under six years of age have been especially prone, but so have some adolescents. Six children under the age of three have already died.

The task

Analyse the problem according to the sequence of the nine epidemiological questions and give a short answer to each question. If necessary, indicate the kind of additional information you might want.

FINAL TEST

You can use the same questions as in the three teaching games to give the participants their final test. Discuss the correct answers afterwards. If, and only if, you did a test at the beginning can the advancement of the participants' knowledge be measured.

EVALUATION OF THE WORKSHOP

Pin on the board the following cards:

What was positive?	What was negative?	Suggestions

The participants write down their comments on cards and put them on the respective topics (methodology, contents, organization, materials, work environment, etc.). Afterwards, the facilitator reads them aloud.

ADDITIONAL TRAINING MODULES

The following modules A4 and A5 are meant to reinforce the health workers' ability to apply epidemiological tools and thinking to their work.

MODULE A4. WHO IS AFFECTED? (The Risk Approach)

1. The facilitator reminds the participants of the definition of 'risk group' and 'risk factors' (see Module 2, Question 5, 'Who is affected?'). This can be accomplished by means of a didactic game (Appendixes A.3, in which questions on the risk approach are used) or by a general discussion.

2. The participants split into smaller groups and are shown the following figures for analysis (copied from Appendix A.1).

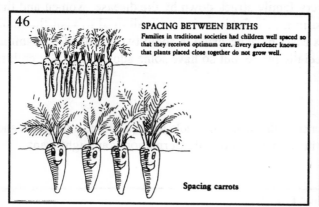

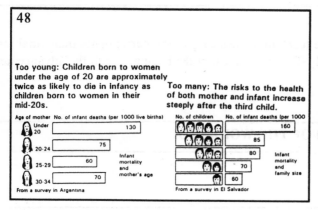

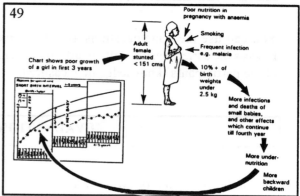

Source: Morley and Lovel 1986.

3. The participants must now do the following:
(a) Identify the risk factors (in each of them)
(b) Match the risk factors with the corresponding diseases from the examples in the drawing.
(c) Draw conclusions from each of them.

4. Answer the following questions:
(a) Which risk factors correspond with which disease(s)? Can you identify them?
(b) Drawing 51 shows a difficult delivery. What kind of risk factors can cause problems at birth?

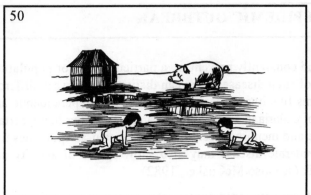

50

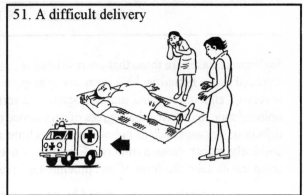

51. A difficult delivery

5.   The participants must (a) draw up a list of health problems and associated risk factors in their own communities, and (b) arrange them in the following table:

Health problem	Risk factor	How can we identify people at risk?

For example: childhood malnutrition, problems during pregnancy and delivery, caries (cavities), diarrhoeal diseases (see Module A1).

6.   Each group chooses one of the examples shown in the pictures and discussed during the morning session. (Groups can now be mixed, according to the areas of interest of respective participants.)

7.   Discuss the possible interventions in relation to the health problem.

8.   Fill in the following table:

Health problem...................................... Risk factors......................................			
ACTIVITY	OBJECTIVE	TARGET	ASSUMPTIONS/CONDITIONS

9.   Hold a plenary session so that each group can present its own results.

MODULE A5. AN EPIDEMIC OUTBREAK

Endemic diseases are those that are restricted to, and constantly present in, a particular area or population. Typhoid fever, hepatitis, kala–azar are examples of such diseases. One can distinguish between different levels of endemicity, and malarialogists use terms like hypoendemic, mesoendemic, hyperendemic and holoendemic to describe the degrees of prevalence of malaria in a particular area. On the other hand, certain infectious diseases such as bubonic plague, cholera and meningococcal meningitis occur as epidemics that suddenly affect great numbers of people. An endemic disease may also show spikes of activity and temporarily take the form of an epidemic outbreak (see also McCusker, 1982)

An epidemic is characterized by an unusual and very rapid numerical increase in a specific disease or health-related event among many individuals in a given community or district, well in excess of what could normally be expected. The number of cases indicating the presence of an epidemic varies according to the agent involved, the population affected, and the time and place of occurrence.

In point-source epidemics, an explosive increase in the number of cases occurs because of the exposure of many individuals susceptible to a particular pathogenic agent or toxin. In a contagious disease epidemic, the propagation of the disease is often less abrupt. The term epidemic may be applied to any sudden increase in the incidence rate of an infectious or noninfectious disease among individuals in a particular area.

The following steps should be taken when investigating a suspected epidemic outbreak:

---

1. Ascertain the correctness of the diagnosis.

2. If warranted, confirm the existence of the epidemic.

3. Identify the affected persons and look for additional cases.

4. Determine who in the population is more particularly at risk.

5. Try to ascertain the cause and the scope of the epidemic (why and how it spread and whether there is a risk of spreading into other as yet unaffected areas).

6. Initiate the necessary steps to bring the epidemic under control. This entails case management (treatment), stringent control and containment measures, strict monitoring, writing a report.

7. Confirm by experimental methods the nature of the causal agent of the disease as well as the propagation mode of the epidemic.

Display the above on a flip chart or on a wall sheet.

Case study

The following case study, 'Outbreak of an unidentified diarrhoeal disease' is to be copied and distributed to the participants to enable them to see how the 'seven investigative steps' are applied in reality. Our example is based on an actual case observed and documented by A. and W. Seidel.

Outbreak of an unidentified diarrhoeal disease

Health Centre D is the referral centre for three administrative units (D, B and T), with 150 villages and total population of 100,000 (Fig. 1). There are also two dispensaries. The total number of medical personnel in the zone is 18. The population lives mainly from subsistence farming. Drinking-water is drawn from shallow wells and water holes.

On 10 August, 1986, at the height of the rainy season, the District Medical Officer is informed by the Zonal Administrative Officer of the outbreak of an unidentified diarrhoeal disease with often fatal outcome in a village 45 kilometres away (150 households, total population of 1,700). A visit to the village the next day reveals the following:

- Nine cases have been observed since the beginning of the preceding month (July). All affected persons suffer from diarrhoea accompanied by vomiting, but not fever; they eventually lapse into coma.
- Only two dehydrated patients are found in the village during the field trip: a young adult who is already recovering and symptom-free, and a malnourished four-year-old child.

As there is no further evidence of an epidemic outbreak, the Community Health Worker and the Village Health Committee are instructed:

- to report any further fatal cases immediately
- to apply strictly the standard Oral Rehydration Treatment (ORT) to diarrhoeal cases
- to give early antidiarrhoeal treatment
- to promote latrine construction.

Thirteen days later, on 23 August, the Zonal Administrative Officer informs the District Medical Officer that six deaths have occurred in the village of unit B and that medical intervention is urgently needed. However, during the course of a visit by medical personnel the very same day, the Village Health Centre can present the visitors with only a six-year-old girl showing clinical signs of diarrhoea and dehydration and in need of i.v. treatment. It is only by accident that another 14-year-old girl, dehydrated and already in a coma, is found during the village inspection tour.

First group exercise

Answer the following questions

1. What kind of disease outbreak is likely in this case?
2. What kind of information would you seek and what investigative procedure ('steps') would you follow before settling on a course of action?
3. How long could you wait in this situation before initiating the course of action you have decided on?

On 23 August, the day of the medical inspection, a treatment centre is established in the village school building. It is staffed by a health-centre nurse and the Community Health Worker. In addition:

- all wells are inspected and chlorinated
- three teams visit every household to look for as yet uncovered cases and distribute sulfadoxine tablets to all household members; households lacking an acceptable toilet are asked to install one the very same day
- the following day, 24 August, is declared 'village-cleaning-day' and thorough cleaning of the village takes place under the supervision of the District Medical Officer
- no open-air market is held
- an epidemiological curve is established. It is based on the household information collected (Fig. 2).

On 24 August, one new case, and on 25 August, two new cases are detected and treated. No further cases are found after that date. Three weeks later, the National Laboratory is able to confirm the diagnosis serologically: Vibrio Cholerae, biotype El Tor, serotype Ogawa.

Second group exercise

1. Discuss the epidemiological curve and the measures taken.
2. Do you think the drug prophylaxis alone brought about the end of the epidemic or were there other factors involved?
3. What percentage of the population do you think may develop the disease?

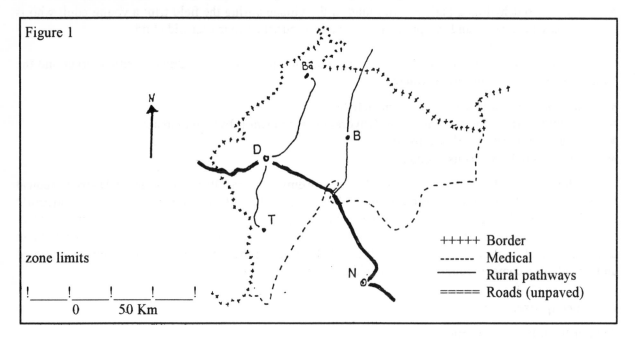

Figure 1

N

zone limits

!____!____!____!____!____!
0   5.0 Km

+++++ Border
------- Medical
——— Rural pathways
===== Roads (unpaved)

Figure 2
Situation on 25 August, 1986

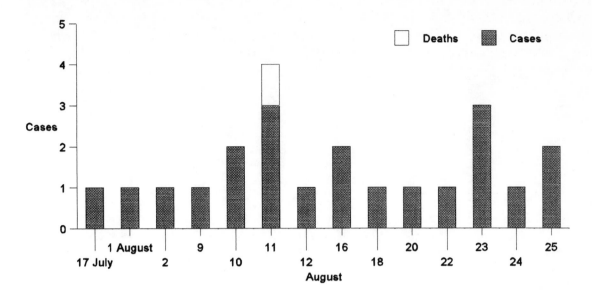

PART B

PART B

ANALYSIS OF HEALTH SERVICES AND LOCAL PLANNING

Preparation and Schedule of the Workshop

The following parts of this volume should be copied and handed over either to each participant or to each group, during the workshop:

TO BE COPIED FOR EACH PARTICIPANT
1. Appendix B.1, B.4 and B.5
2. Text on pp. 54-56
3. Table of activities, p. 72
4. Module B.4 and B.5 (if these are dealt with)

TO BE COPIED FOR EACH GROUP
1. The questions for the teaching games, each one written out on a separate card (Appendix B.3)
2. The rules and how to play the games (Appendix B.3)

The following tables should be written on a large sheet of paper, which will be pinned during the workshop on to Styrofoam plates fastened to the wall.

TABLES SHOULD BE ENLARGED AND WRITTEN ON LARGE SHEETS OF PAPER
1. The timetable of the workshop
2. Start, breaks and end of each working day
3. The 9 questions related to classical epidemiology and health care epidemiology (p. 58)
4. The Management cycle (p. 57)
5. 'How can we measure equity in our district?' (p. 63)
6. Table on indicators (p. 133 in Appendix B.1)
7. Which seasonal variations (p.61)

The workshop is organized exactly as in Part A, that is to say there will be four sessions each day lasting between one-and-a-half and two hours, two sessions in the morning, two in the afternoon with an occasional additional session in the evening. Each session is followed by a break. The topics to be covered and the tasks to be performed during the course of each session should have been determined in advance. It is important, however, to remain flexible and to adapt the progress of the workshop to the specific requirements of a given group of participants. If long discussions arise on one topic, it may prove necessary to halt an unfinished session and to hold an additional one in the evening. As the rate of progress of the workshop depends on local circumstances, we suggest that the following is taken to be only a general guide to the distribution of the topics to be covered during the week:

THE SIX-DAY WORKSHOP

Day No	1	2	3	4	5	6
MORNING (2 sessions)	Module B1	Module B1 (cont'd)	Module B2	Module B2 (cont'd)	Module B2 Management Exercises	Module B2 (cont'd)
AFTERNOON (2 sessions)	Module B1 (cont'd)	Module B1 (cont'd)	Module B2 (cont'd)	Module B2 (cont'd)	Module B2 (cont'd)	Final test and evaluation of the workshop

Additional one-to-three-day modules

Module B3   Improving technical work at local level

Module B4   Assessing quality of service

Module B5   Improving acceptance through recognition of local cultural factors

Module B6   Making a census

Structure of the Workshop on Local Programming

TOPIC	OBJECTIVES	PROCEDURE	MATERIALS	TIME[1]
MODULE B1				
Introduction to the district concept Introduction to the management cycle	To know the district health system concept To know the components of the management cycle and their definitions	Text reading Discussion Presentation and discussion	Documents on district health concept (WHO–PAHO) Card with the management cycle	1 session
Q.1 Main health problems	To apply the nine epidemiological questions to health-service problems and to analyse their causes	Brainstorming on health problems. Prioritizing the problems on the matrix (plenary)	Cards, markers, boards. Prioritization matrix	1 session
Q.2 What is the magnitude of the problems?	To know the most important indicators	Reading of text on indicators Teaching games Comparative data	Appendices B1, B4, B5 Teaching games with set of questions	2 sessions
Q.3 When do the problems or health events increase?	To understand the seasonal variation of health-service problems	Group work on the matrix Diagram on monitoring of coverage	Squared paper Chart with the matrix on styrofoam board	1 session
Q.4 and Q.5 Where and whom do the health problems affect?	To analyse the geographical variation of the problems	Drawing simplified maps Proportion Calculation	Copies with tasks, paper, markers	1 session
Q.6 Why do the problems occur?	To analyse the causes of health services problems	Option A: Causation Tree Option B: Use of the matrix	Matrix on a card	2 sessions

---

[1]   A session corresponds to 90 minutes

TOPIC	OBJECTIVES	PROCEDURE	MATERIALS	TIME[1]
MODULE B.2				
Introduction to the Matrix	To know a simple planning tool, and apply it to the participants' own situation	Plenary session: Facilitator presents an example on the matrix Reading of instructions and how to apply them Group work Information market	Matrix Matrix	2 sessions 8 to 12 sessions

MODULE B1. ANALYSIS OF HEALTH–SERVICE PROBLEMS

1. *Introduction to the district health concept*

Discuss the concept as well as the potentials and pitfalls of the district health system. (Before or after the discussion the groups can read the following documents about the district health system and extract the main characteristics of the concept. They can write it on cards and pin these on the board.)

A district health system based on primary health care is a more or less self-contained segment of the national health system. It comprises first and foremost a well-defined population, living within a clearly delineated administrative and geographical area, whether urban or rural. It includes all institutions and individuals providing health care in the district, whether governmental, social security, non-governmental, private, or traditional. A district health system therefore consists of a large variety of interrelated elements that contribute to health in related sectors. It includes self-care and all health-care workers and facilities, up to and including the hospital at the first referral level, as well as the appropriate laboratory and other diagnostic and logistic support services. Its component elements need to be well coordinated by elements and institutions into a fully comprehensive range of promotional, preventive, curative, and rehabilitative activities.

(WHO 1988)

The health sector should monitor, organize, and participate in the processes of local development. Therefore, the definition of local health systems (district health systems) according to the health sector, should facilitate a greater adaptation and enhanced capacity to respond to changing and specific requirements of the population groups affected by common socio-economic, environmental, and epidemiological problems. As a result, there are a number of elements specific to the health sector that can be observed in two supplementary areas: the reorganization and reorientation of the sector's structure based on the processes of decentralization; and reorganization of the services network within a defined population area.

continued

---

[1] A session corresponds to 90 minutes

A local health system should have an office responsible for the administration of health actions in a given population area. This implies an ability to manage some resources directly and to coordinate the entire social infrastructure devoted to health, based on a geographical area, on a scale capable of resolving a significant number of health problems of individuals, families, social groups, communities, and environment, and also to facilitate social participation and coordination with national health systems in order to strengthen and redirect these systems.

The administrative level should, in turn, take on the responsibility for management of all of the existing resources (hospitals, health centres and posts, water supply systems and other sanitation services and extrasectorial resources) in a specified population area so as to achieve optimum use of these resources and to ensure their conformance to local reality. As part of this responsibility, it is fundamental that a relationship be established with the population based on mutual responsibilities to face the challenge of ensuring good health.

This reciprocal relationship should be evident in all aspects of individual and collective health, policy- making in the setting of priorities, origin and distribution of resources, programming, implementation, and evaluation, as well as in relation to individual and group behaviour regarding the health–disease process. To the extent that there is a precise definition of the population and the territory to be covered, it becomes possible to evaluate the actions carried out or that need to be taken to respond to local health needs.

Local health systems should be seen as the basic organization units of a fully articulated overall network: the national health system. Local health systems are the focal points of peripheral planning and management of health services; they fall under the integrative and normative influence of the health system's national coordinating structure, where overall policy is made, and also where systems of logistical, technical, and administrative support required for the programme implementation and provision of services at the local level are defined. Within this national scheme, local health systems can become the basis for defining regionalized health systems.

Considering the above, local health systems need to take into account the political administrative structure of a country, be defined to specific population areas; take into account all available resources in the area of health and social development; respond to processes of state and health sector decentralization, to population needs, to the structure of the health services network, and be organized so as to facilitate comprehensive administration.

A local health system should be based on an analysis of the health situation, including knowledge of the needs, and identifying and qualifying conditions of risk so as to orient the definition of priorities, organization, and the use of available resources.

Taking into account the need to continue and promote the development of innovative models of health service at the level of local health systems, the process of research on, and assessment of health services should be fundamental in the reorganization and reorientation of the health sector from the beginning.

continued

The fundamental aspects of local health systems development include:

- Decentralization/deconcentration

- Community participation/social participation

- Intersectoral coordination

- Adjustment of financing mechanisms

- Development of new care models

- Integration of prevention and control programmes

- Strengthening of managerial capacity

- Training of the work force in health

- Research

(PAHO/WHO 1992)

2.   *Introduction to the management cycle*

1.   Pin a large sheet of paper showing the management cycle on to the Styrofoam.

2.   Remind participants of what has been done in Part A of the workshop, and explain what is going to be done now (pin short memos beside the corresponding boxes).

(a)   Analysis of the present situation – that is, what has been done in Part A about health problems – by answering the nine epidemiological questions applied to the health-service problems.

(b)   Appraisal of district priorities: has it been covered in Part A regarding health problems? This has to be carried out regarding health-service problems as well.

(c)   Setting objectives and targets: this should be covered in different modules of Part B of this workshop as well.

(d)   District action programme to improve health services and to design joint actions (this task will be carried out in Module B2).

(e)   Brief discussion of the definition of monitoring and evaluation.

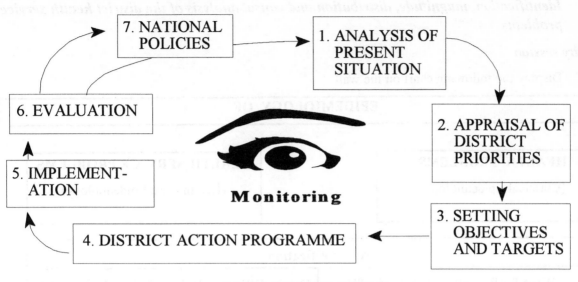

MANAGEMENT CYCLE

MONITORING	EVALUATION
The continuous measurement and observation of the performance of the health service or health programme to see that it is proceeding according to the proposed plans and objectives.	The repeated measurement of the same phenomena (e.g. every year).

3. *Identification, magnitude, distribution and causal analysis of the district health service problems*

Plenary session

1. Display the following chart on the wall

EPIDEMIOLOGY OF

HEALTH PROBLEMS (Classical Epidemiology)	HEALTH-SERVICE PROBLEMS (Health Care Epidemiology)

A. Identification			
Q.1	WHAT ARE THE MAIN HEALTH PROBLEMS?	Q.1	WHAT ARE THE MAIN PROBLEMS OF THE HEALTH SERVICES?
B. Magnitude and Distribution			
Q.2	How many?	Q.2	How many problems?
Q.3	When do cases occur?	Q.3	When do problems increase?
Q.4	Where do cases occur?	Q.4	Where do problems arise?
Q.5	Who is affected?	Q.5	Who is affected?
C: Analysis			
Q.6	Why?	Q.6	Why?
D. Measures taken			
Q.7	Measures taken to cope with the problem	Q.7	Measures taken to cope with the problem
Q.8	Results? Difficulties?	Q.8	Results? Difficulties?
Q.9	What else can be done?	Q.9	What else can be done?

2. Explain that the health service's problems can be assessed by means of the nine epidemiological questions.

3. Read aloud the questions on the right hand side of the diagram and explain that questions Q.1 to Q.6 will be dealt with in Module B1 and questions Q.7 to Q.9 in Module B2.

| Q.1 | What are the main problems of the health services in our district? |

Group exercise and plenary session (45 minutes)

1.   Put to the participants the following questions:

'What are the main problems related to the health services in your area?'

Each participant lists one to three problems on one to three different charts which are gathered and pinned on the Styrofoam covered wall.

2.   With prior consent of the group, only those charts with different problems written on them are to be retained.

3.   Each group pins the cards on the wall sheet.

4.   In a plenary session, the first eight health problems elaborated by the groups are copied in the first column of the priority-setting matrix (see table below).

5.   All participants prioritize the health-services' problems giving ten points in each column (see explanation on page 24).

6.   Discuss the problem prioritized with participants.

PRIORITIZATION OF HEALTH-SERVICES' PROBLEMS

PROBLEM	Negative impact on the population's health[1]	How far is it from the expected results[2]	Is it considered as a problem by the community[3]	Possibilities of improvement at district level[4]	TOTAL

---

[1]   Has this problem direct consequences on the population's health? (E.g.: low coverage of sanitation programmes)

[2]   Is it a severe problem? (E.g.: Immunization coverage=20% is too far from the expected coverage)

[3]   Does the community perceive shortage of personnel, low converage of immunization, etc. as problems?

[4]   Possibilities of improving at local level, in terms of costs and feasibility of control.

Part B

Indicators for the assessment of health services

Q.2	How many health-service problems exist? Session on indicators

Plenary session

1. Each participant receives a copy of Appendix B.1. 'Indicators for district health systems'. (If possible, this handout should have been given to the participants in advance)

2. The facilitator explains briefly what an indicator is (first part of Appendix B.1), and then the framework of the indicators.

Group exercise

3. The participants get 90 minutes to read Appendix B.1 through, together or individually. Another possibility is to present first the matrix of health indicators and afterwards do the exercise in Appendix B.5.

4. Afterwards, the participants play, in their groups, the first teaching game. This lasts about 45 minutes (rules and instructions are to be found in Appendix B.3).

5. After the game, facilitators discuss open questions which arose during the game.

    If necessary, the facilitator provides the correct answers for each question. (This can also be done in a plenary session.)

6. Facilitators stress the fact that we have now learned an important tool for the assessment of different aspects of the health services. However,

•   Indicators measure only very specific components; thus several indicators are needed for the assessment of different aspects of the health system

•   The indicators mentioned in Appendix 1 are not the only ones. The list provides important examples and a quite comprehensive framework. Within the same framework, additional indicators can be developed according to the health services' specific needs. Examples: availability of additional funds, availability of standard equipment, regularity of supervision, functioning of community health committees; acceptance of family planning devices (see part C of Appendix B.1).

7. Group exercise on the use of indicators in a model district (Appendix B5)

Plenary session

8. Priority setting of health-service problems (see matrix) using the same methodologies as in part A of this manual.

Q.3	When do the problems increase?

Group exercise

1. Each group takes some problems identified in their district in one of the main areas: availability (e.g. of VHW[1]); process (e.g. use of services, utilization of resources); output (coverage, efficiency) and outcome (effectiveness).

2. Answer the following questions and present the results on a new wall-chart:

Which seasonal variations of your health services' indicators will probably occur?				
Write down additional indicators that may show seasonal variations. (Write comments on additional charts and pin them up in the last column.)				
Indicator	Increased (I) or decreased (D) during:			
	dry season	wet season	others (specify)	comments
Availability of VHW[1]				
Use of services				
• vaccination coverage				
• antenatal care coverage				
• weight monitoring				
Productivity of staff				
Efficiency of staff				
Effectiveness of the service				

Group exercise (Variation of coverage over the year)

(a) Coverage

Example:

$$\text{Annual obstetric coverage in a given district} = \frac{\text{Number of deliveries attended by a qualified midwife or obstetrician}}{\text{expected number of deliveries during the year in a given district}} \times 100$$

Many health programmes are assigned specific targets that must be met in a year's time. This may pertain to the number of children to be vaccinated, the number of pregnancies to be followed, the number of under-fives for whom growth must be monitored, etc.

---

[1] VHW= Village Health Worker

61

Part B

The kind of diagram shown below is frequently used to illustrate a given programme's rate of progress, in this case, measles vaccination coverage. In this case, the target number of children to be immunized against measles is 2,200, which will mean 100% coverage.

What are the main limitations of such an approach? (Discuss particularly the problem of getting reliable data about the number of children to be immunized.)

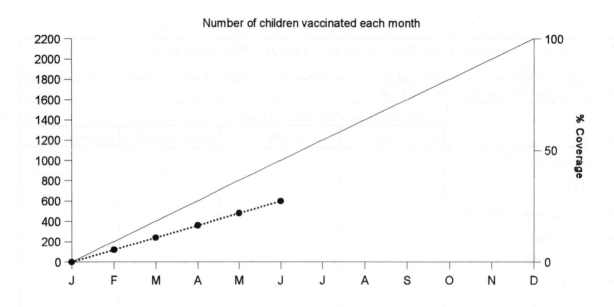

Number of children vaccinated each month

(b)   Use the data below for your coverage diagram.

Expected number of deliveries: 356

Actual deliveries by qualified personnel:

January	10	May	10	September	15
February	15	June	21	October	23
March	20	July	5	November	20
April	16	August 8		December	15

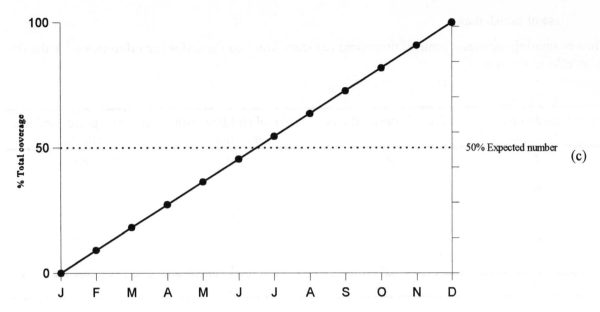

Answer the following questions:

- When tallying up the actual coverage, what problems do you come up with?
- How do you interpret the success of the programme? What has been achieved?

(d)   Discuss the usefulness of these diagrams for the work of their own health team, using examples from the participants' own data (see Appendix B.2, possible solutions).

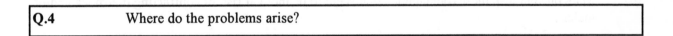

Q.4	Where do the problems arise?

Q.5	Who is concerned?

Group exercise

1.   Each group draws one or two sketch maps of their own work area, ranking the places where the main health-service problems occur (low coverage, low productivity, etc.).

2.   Discussion about possible causes of these differences.

3.   The facilitator pins on the wall sheet (or Styrofoam plate) a chart with the following question:

HOW CAN WE MEASURE EQUITY IN OUR DISTRICT?

The participants are asked to write their answers on cards and pin them up, below the corresponding question. Afterwards, the answers are discussed. (Use a simple operational definition of *equity* which means that all inhabitants should have equal access to and coverage by health services and programmes)

4.   Use of sketch maps

When examining the health centres' outpatient registers, you find the following information for the first six months of the year.

Community	No. of consultations	No. of children with diarrhoea	No. of reported malaria attacks
A	500	30	80
B	90	18	14
C	40	3	6
D	72	7	22
E	33	6	7
TOTAL	735	64	129

(a)   Calculate the number of consultations per person during the first six months of the year. How do you account for the differences between the communities?

(b)   Determine the proportion of children suffering from diarrhoea and that of people with malaria attacks. How do you explain the differences between the communities?

(c)   How would you go about obtaining more accurate data about the greater risk of contracting malaria and/or diarrhoeal diseases that some communities face?

(d)   Mark on your map those communities that seem to be more at risk of contracting diarrhoea and/or malaria.

Q.6	Why does this problem occur?

Group exercise

Option A

1.   Each group takes one of the problems identified in the preceding session and works out a causation tree. This is the graphic representation of a hypothetical model of causes and effects explaining the rate of occurrence of a particular problem. (The procedure is explained in Part A of this manual.)

Possible problems to be analysed could be the following:

*   low vaccination coverage
*   lack of supervision of peripheral services
*   low motivation of VHW (or other personnel)
*   deficient skills of staff in the outpatient department
*   under-use of preventive services

2.   Try to use the indicators for the measurement of different elements within the causation tree.

3. Try to express the indicators in numbers and percentages (using locally available data) and draw conclusions.

Option B

1. Participants fill in charts which they pin on the following table, placed on the Styrofoam plate on the wall.

Problems relating to health services are those they have identified in the previous session or in the first session, and/or they take the examples mentioned above in option A.

Health-services' problems	Indicators to measure the problems	Formula to calculate numerical indicators	Why does the problem arise? (main reasons)

Plenary session

The facilitator presents the planning matrix (see below) and explains the following procedure (if possible, each participant or group should have this text in advance).

MODULE B2. INTRODUCTION TO THE MATRIX

Use of the planning matrix

The planning matrix is a tool which helps to apply in a sequential form the planning process. The structure consists of two different parts:

1. Diagnosis of the present situation

2. Planning of activities to improve the present situation.

Before using the matrix, it is necessary to select the topics that will be analysed in the planning process. The topics are the different subject areas to be included in the process. The success of the work with the matrix depends largely on the correct selection of the topics.

PLANNING MATRIX

ANALYSIS OF THE ACTUAL SITUATION					PROGRAMMING					
ANALYSIS and THEMES to PROGRAMING	ANALYSIS of ACHIEVEMENTS and POTENTIALS	PROBLEM ANALYSIS			Prioritized tasks by sequence and importance	TARGETS (expected results till next evaluation)	RESOURCES		TIME REQUIRED[1] (timetable)	PERSON(S) RESPON-SIBLE
		Problems	Prioritization	Causes			existent	additional		

You can write the timetable (using bar charts) on a separate sheet of paper.

Instructions on how to choose the topics

1. The topics should be based on the analysis of the health problems and health-services' problems (previous modules), and upon the priority matrices.

2. The participants study carefully the list of problems (e.g. in the causal model) putting emphasis on those points which are vulnerable.

3. Group similar problems together, (e.g. institutional structure, functions, procedures, norms, etc. Can be put together under a common title, 'organization of health services').

4. Look for possible topics to be included and the main aspects that may have been overlooked by the participants (see later).

After selecting the topics, it is very important to define the meaning of different technical terms, in order to unify the definitions to be used by the participants.

For example: What is 'organisation'? What is 'quality of care'? Write the definitions down.

The definition of the terminology avoids misunderstandings in the following steps of the planning matrix.

The matrix must be used in a dynamic way, moving forwards and backwards, and never as a rigid diagram.

List of possible topics:

	Problems in:
Organization of health services	Admission for consultation Referral system Comprehensive care Organizational structure, norms and rules, functions, procedures Management lines
Management	Information systems Quality of care Health financing Co–ordination between/within institutions
Supervision and monitoring	Training Evaluation Supervision and training of midwives, nurses, health auxiliaries, village health workers, and others
Community participation	Participation in: Planning Decision making Implementation Evaluation
Contents of the programmes	Water and sanitation Maternal and child health Nutrition Treatment of frequent diseases Control of endemic diseases Health education Essential drugs Immunization

Analysis of the present situation

This part presents an analysis of the health service, its achievements and potentials. This can be used as a basis for identifying the main problems and their possible causes.

Analysis of achievements and potentials (Question 7).
This analysis describes the current situation (e.g. 5 training courses have been carried out in the last year), and the resources used (e.g. training institutions involved, different methodologies successfully used, etc.).

Analysis of problems
According to the results of Module B1, we do need to have a list of problems, among which we underline the main problem included in the topics.

Prioritization
If the prioritization of the problems has not been done before (Module B1), it is necessary now to select the main problems, taking into account the level of susceptibility to intervention (e.g. the workers who received the training courses do not put into practice their newly acquired knowledge).

Causes

For each problem identified as a priority, it is necessary to describe the possible causes, choosing particularly problems which provide possibilities of action.

Here, one can use the 'problem tree' because it is a technique which explains, in a hypothetical form, possible relationships between factors associated with the problem.

It is very important to make a good analysis of the possible causes for each priority problem, for this is the basis for making up a good plan.

In simple words, we can define the relationship between the third level of problems in the first part of the matrix as follows:

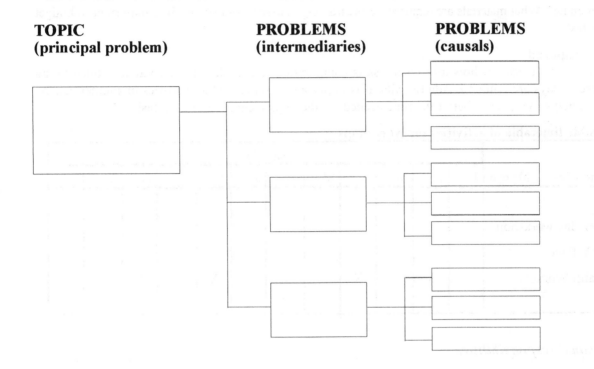

| TOPIC (principal problem) | PROBLEMS (intermediaries) | PROBLEMS (causals) |

Actions

Programme planning

This refers to the measures to be taken in order to improve the 'present situation'. The programme planning includes definition of tasks, targets, resources required, time required to implement the planned activities, and, last but not least, the persons responsible for each task.

Tasks by sequence and importance

Firstly, it is necessary to specify in chronological order the activities to be carried out in order to improve the 'present situation'. The emphasis should be on some specific actions, e.g. 'to train village health workers', and should include the following sub-activities, which are enumerated:

1.1   to identify training needs

1.2   to design the content of the workshop

1.3   to define the number of participants, duration of the course, and profile of the participants.

The task should be written down in infinitive verbs indicating the actions which have to be done. Sometimes, the tasks are not put in a chronological sequence, but in the order of importance regarding their implementation.

Targets

For each task, a target has to be set. A target is a concrete objective which we would like to achieve in a given time. For example: to run 4 training courses before December. Each course lasts 5 days, and it is desirable that courses are held every two months.

Resources required

It is necessary to detail the resources needed for the implementation of the plan, specifying the existing resources and the additional ones required. For example: How many nurses are needed in a PHC programme? What materials are required for the training course? And so on. It is important to budget each task.

Time required

It is necessary to specify how long each task is going to take, e.g. to design the content of the training course, 5 days are required. Additionally, it is important to schedule the activities in another matrix, as this helps to visualize better the time needed for the implementation of each task.

Possible timetable of activities for workshops

Activities Month	J	F	M	A	M	J	J	A	S	O	N	D
Two–day workshop for Village Health Workers		X		X		X		X		X		

Persons' responsibilities

It is necessary to define who is responsible for carrying out each task or monitoring if it has been done. It is important to write down the names and departments that will carry out or monitor the task.

Group exercise

(a)   Firstly, participants work on the 'problem analysis', using the results of Module B1, particularly the 'problem tree'.

(b)   The groups present their results using a method called 'information market'. Its rules should be written on a large piece of paper and shown to the participants.

Rules for the information market

1. The text on the board illustrates the results of the group discussions.

    They are self explanatory, which means that you can understand them without additional comments.

2. You are asked to look at the posters elaborated by other groups and to write down your comments and suggestions on the charts. Pin the charts on the posters.

3. The groups meet again and modify their posters according to the comments received.

(c) After participants have incorporated the suggestions from the 'information market'' into their own work, the next step is to continue with the 'planning of activities', the second part of the matrix.

(d) The groups again interchange suggestions and comments by observing the other groups' posters, and using the 'information market' method.

(e) Finally, the groups present the programme of activities to be carried out in the time previously determined (e.g. for one year).

Evaluation of the workshop

The evaluation of the workshop will be done in the same way as in Part A.

MODULE B3. IMPROVING TECHNICAL WORK AT LOCAL LEVEL

In this module, the group work should be done by the participants from the same institution and belonging to the same health team.

Group exercise

General considerations

Applying simple techniques and approaches for organizing the work of the basic health units around the health needs of the population in their assigned area could bring about a substantial improvement in coverage, effectiveness and motivation. Examples of such techniques and approaches are listed hereafter (the facilitator may want to write an abbreviated form of the following table on a wall paper/flip chart).

IMPROVING TECHNICAL WORK AT LOCAL LEVEL

This can be achieved by:

---

1. **A rational work organization,** including:

    (a)   *technical meetings* of the whole team on a regular basis in order to discuss health and health-service problems, and to establish programmes and evaluate them

    (b)   making *weekly work plans* for each staff member, including regular work in the community

    (c)   delineation of *shared objectives* regarding improvement of community health, promotion of health and community development

2. **The use of epidemiological tools** such as:

    (a)   the information produced in the unit itself for programming, monitoring and evaluation, e.g. estimating *coverage* achieved and *targeting further coverage*

    (b)   *maps* for establishing work progress, localizing risk areas and dividing the catchment area * into subsectors

3. **Additional data collection** through:

    (a)   taking a simple *census* (counting the houses and individuals in the community)

    (b)   finding out about health interests and activities of community organizations

    (c)   reports from donor agencies, ministries, etc.

4. **Improvement of curative care** by:

    (a)   ensuring patients' continuity of care by the same staff members

    (b)   designing a screening system in the outpatient clinic for the detection of patients in need of special attention (patients from broken families, high-risk communities, etc.)

---

1. Start a discussion about the following points:

(a)   Are these suggestions realistic for your own health team?

(b)   What has already been done? Where and when can the improvements be done? If and only if possible, determine dates for regular technical meetings of the team, define objectives, and establish flexible work plans.

2. Use the planning matrix for the activities in your own area.

Time allocation

Your workplace is a health unit located in a rural district and staffed with one physician, two auxiliary nurses, one laboratory technician and one clerk. Each of them works six hours a day, six days a week.

As there is no job description for these five people, you are to establish a weekly working plan. The drawings you will see show the activities the health team has identified as important.

---

*   Catchment area: the geographical area from which the people attending a particular health facility come (Vaughan and Morrow 1989)

(a)   Use the table immediately below ('List of activities according to time requirements') to order the activities in decreasing order of implementation time: the most time-consuming ones at the top, those requiring the least time at the bottom, the others in between.

The cards bearing the drawings of those activities that are not to be carried out by this particular health unit are not to be listed in the table, but must remain visibly displayed. Should some activities be missing, write their names on separate cards and include them in the list.

(b)   Once you have ordered the drawings and entered (in the same order) in the table the names of the activities they represent, write on the cards and in the table (next to the relevant activity) the number of working hours per activity per week. If the same activity has to be performed by several staff members separately, the total time needed for it must be entered. If a particular activity is performed only once or twice a month, write this down as well.

(c)   Discuss the suitability of this exercise for your own health unit and mark the cards depicting those activities which should be emphasized in your own work.

LIST OF ACTIVITIES ACCORDING TO TIME REQUIREMENTS		
physician	auxiliary nurse	laboratory technician

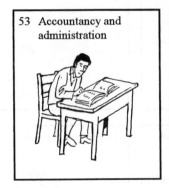

53 Accountancy and administration

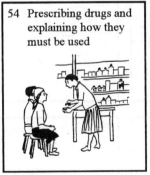

54 Prescribing drugs and explaining how they must be used

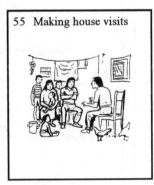

55 Making house visits

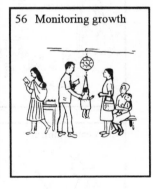

56 Monitoring growth

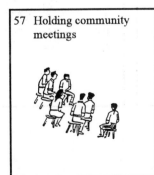

57 Holding community meetings

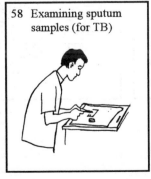

58 Examining sputum samples (for TB)

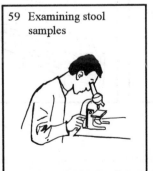

59 Examining stool samples

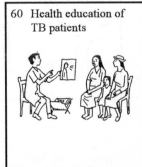

60 Health education of TB patients

61 Gathering medicinal plants	62 Collecting natural medicinal products	63 Immunization	64 Curative medicine
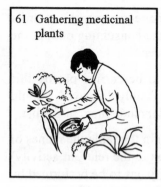	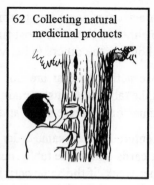	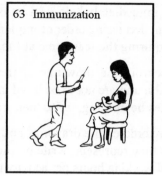	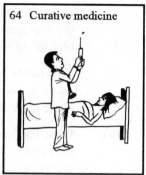
65 Rehabilitation	66 Provision of drinking water	67 Information on nutrition	68 Breast-feeding
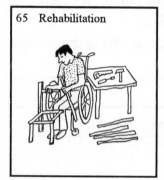	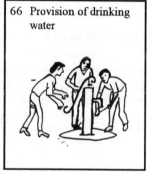	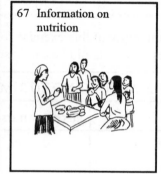	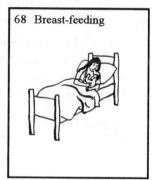
69 Food hygiene	70 Water hygiene	71 Improvement of housing	72 Improvement of latrines
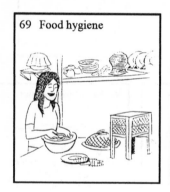	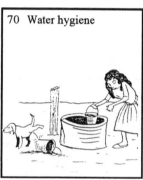	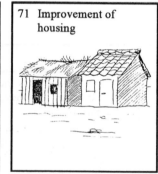	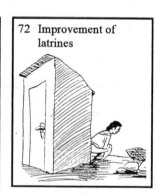
73 Vector control	74 Malaria prophylaxis	75 Improving community development	76 Treating the sick
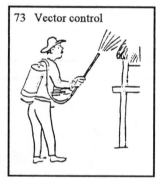	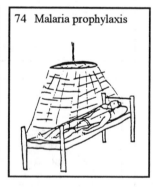	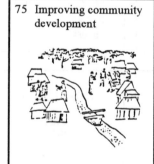	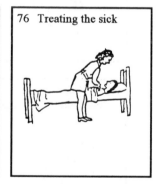

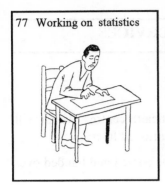

77 Working on statistics

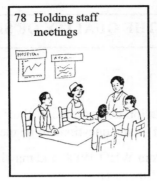

78 Holding staff meetings

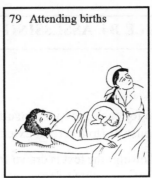

79 Attending births

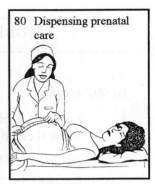

80 Dispensing prenatal care

Finding out about the interests and activities of community organizations

The communication between community and health workers can be improved when these take part in community meetings and assemblies. Attending these is the best way to find out what is 'going on', whether people are or can be motivated to participate in the planning and implementation of public health measures, such as keeping community grounds and latrines clean, providing containers or digging holes for the garbage, and so forth.

1.   Put the drawings into an order that permits you to identify the sequence of planning, implementing, reporting, reassessing.

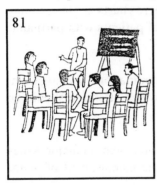

81

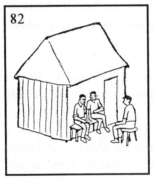

82

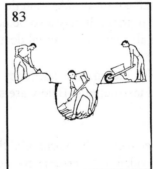

83

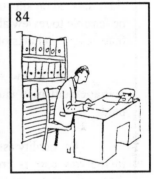

84

MODULE B4. ASSESSING THE QUALITY OF SERVICES

Group work

1. Have available for each group a consultation book of one of their health centres, which will allow them to answer (to a certain extent) some questions to be mentioned later.

2. Explain the following (the text is drawn from WHO 1988, and may be copied and handed over to the participants or written down on a flipchart):

Quality in health *is the degree to which resources for health care* or the services included in health care *correspond to specific standards*. All hospitals, health centres and other health units should audit the quality of services provided, at least quarterly. The audit should be carried out by a committee chaired by the officer in charge and may include all staff. A record of the findings should be made for the information of staff who might not have attended the session, and for future reference.

The assessment is based on a *review of charts* and *case notes* for various services, such as antenatal care, child welfare, family planning and in-patients. It is best to review the charts of one kind of service at a time. Charts for review are *selected by some quasi-randomised methods*, e.g. every fifth chart decided on site, taking into consideration the total number of charts. Where charts are few, it may be feasible to review all of them. It may also be decided to review all charts of patients with particular features, e.g. charts of all cases of maternal death.

The review will include the adequacy of the clinical history, examination, investigation, management plan and instructions. Below are some examples of areas to which attention should be paid.

For quality assessment to be meaningful there should be broad prior agreement on major issues in the way care is provided, e.g., criteria for admissions to hospital and the management of major diseases. For example, criteria for admission to hospital might include:

i)   severe anaemia

ii)   persistent fever over 101° (=38.3°C)

iii) abnormal findings in CSF (Cerebrospinal Fluid)

iv)   blood pressure readings under 80 or over 200 and/or less than 60 or greater than 120.

v)   onset of unconsciousness or disorientation

vi)   active bleeding

vii) chest pain and/or signs of acute ischemia

viii) wound or surgical emergency

ix)   obstetric problems, including obstructed labour.

---

3. Questions to be presented to the participants with regard to the consultation book:

MCH programme

(a) Are the schedules of the MCH clinics followed, for example the provision of health education?

(b) Were the minimum prescribed procedures, e.g. BP, urine, HB checks, followed?

(c) Was there adequate follow-up of abnormal findings, such as low haemoglobin or high BP?

(d) Were high-risk patients identified early?

(e) Was the diagnosis and treatment of the illness adequate?

(f) If drugs were prescribed, were they appropriate to the condition?

(g) Were the potential side effects of drugs monitored as necessary?

(h) Is the charting adequate? For example, is the chart legible and key data items such as laboratory results, drugs, progress notes, easy to find?

Any other specific irregularities within individual records which may require further action should be noted.

The review will indicate the level of skills and knowledge of the staff, as well as gaps and lapses in the delivery of services. The information is invaluable for further improvements.

3. Another way of assessing quality is the interview survey among outpatients and/or hospital inpatients about their perceptions of quality of care, friendliness of staff, cleanliness of the building etc. The groups work out a questionnaire for patients' interviews.

MODULE B5. IMPROVING ACCEPTANCE THROUGH RECOGNITION OF LOCAL CULTURAL FACTORS (CULTURAL ACCESSIBILITY)

Group exercise

Have the following text copied and handed over to the participants. The group reads the text together and answers the questions.

---

1.   *Case study in a rural community*

A case study found that most dwellers in the village of Baguineda appreciate folk medicine, modern medicine and Islamic medicine, and that healer shopping (i.e. the multiple use of different sources of health care) is a characteristic of health care choice. Yet people's behaviour in case of illness depends not only on cultural norms and education, but also on the economic situation of the family.

Self-care is generally the first step in the search for the treatment of mild and common symptoms. If this fails, the patient seeks professional advice:

*   in severe, acute cases of natural illness modern medicine is preferred because the outcome of treatment is expected to be quicker, but high costs prevent many patients from utilizing this treatment.

*   folk medicine is considered to be effective, but the patient has to use several remedies over long periods and the treatment has to be repeated from time to time. However, this treatment is available to everyone and frequently at low prices; even payment in kind is accepted.

*   a quick and unusual development of illness will often be associated with black magic or sorcery and thus needs treatment by specialists in the popular medicine sector.

The study indicates that the local population's concepts of and behaviour towards illness are composed of various elements derived from traditional and modern cultural influences. Beside the problems of economic accessibility of health services, the acceptance of effective modern medical treatment may also be hindered by differences in people's concepts of the causes of illness. Due to misunderstandings and communication gaps between villagers and health professionals there exist contrasting conceptions of illness and treatment options which tend to demoralize local communities instead of helping them.

The study concludes that analysis of these differences and problems, conducted with community representatives, is indispensable in the process of planning and implementing health programmes. This does not imply the rejection of traditional medical practices; on the contrary, folk healers should be recognized at the same time as being an integral component of the village health system.

---

2.   *Discussion in group work*

(a)   Discuss the following questions:

*   are there similar/other problems in your own community that prevent healthy behaviour?

*   provide examples of 'cultural misunderstanding' between health staff and population that result in under-use of health services?

- make a list of subjects in which local people's different concepts of illness present obstacles to the health work in your community.
- are there attitudinal problems of health staff in your service resulting in low acceptance of services?

(b)   Apply the problem-analysis technique ('causation tree') to the problems listed in the discussions of the questions above.

(c)   List possible interventions for solving the problems.

(d)   Rank possible interventions that may enhance communication between health staff and population according to their feasibility.

(e)   Who, apart from health workers, has to be approached for implementing the proposed solutions?

(f)   Make a Plan of Action.

3.   *Each group prepares the presentation to the other groups.*

They can prepare a text to be read, a role play or (if at hand) a play with puppets.

Panel session

4.   *Presentation and discussion of the group work.*

MODULE B6. MAKING A CENSUS

Group exercise

Typical population structure

Generally, local health workers can obtain data on the population size of the catchment area of their health unit from the district health manager or the Ministry of Health. This data is based on a nationwide population census, and estimated anew every year. The typical population structure of a rural district looks something like this:

Age groups (years)	Percentage of total	No. of persons
less than 1	4 %	400
1 – 4	14 %	1400
5–14	26 %	2600
15–44	43 %	4300
45+	13 %	1300
Total	100 %	10,000

Exercise 1

(a)   What changes in the percentages shown above would you expect in an area that sees many of its young couples migrate to the big cities?

(b)   What changes in the percentages shown above would you expect in an area where family planning is successful?

The census

You notice that your health unit, despite much effort, has fallen far short of its vaccination targets. You suspect that the population data is inaccurate and that the number of infants in the area is much lower than shown by the data. So you decide to take your own census.

Its scope can vary. For instance, it might count (a) only households, or (b) only people, but (c) it can also record such characteristics as age, sex, income, etc.

(a)   Counting households

At the local level, counting households may prove fairly easy since community leaders often have lists of all households (or they know them by heart) in their area. It is also important, however, to count those households that are located outside the community (but belong to the catchment area), and/or do not pay taxes, and/or are considered socially marginal, and/or do not belong to the cooperative, etc.

Knowing the total number of households turns out to be particularly useful if an estimate of the average number of persons per household has to be made. To this end, national census data can be used (provided no major changes have occurred since it was taken) as well as data from other comparable communities.

(b)   Counting people

Taking a local census yields more accurate data about the population size. Local health workers, including village health workers, community leaders and other persons working for the community, can be used as census-takers. A list of the total number of households (see above) is necessary. Heads of households may be approached by visiting them at home or during community meetings.

Exercise 2

Design a simple form to be filled in by each household, asking for information on the household's composition (number of people and age groups only).

(c)   Recording other characteristics

Proceed as in (b) but use a more detailed form. This requires better writing skills on the part of the census-takers.

Exercise 3

Design a simple form (to be distributed to each household), where you can record the following information about household members (number of people, age-group, sex, education, occupation).

Exercise 4

1.   Demetria is two years old; her father John, 20, has not completed primary school and works as a landless labourer. How would you code these persons in the form given?

2.   You have just completed the 167 household questionnaires in community X, and are now in possession of information on 1,000 people. What is the average size of household in this community?

3.   The data on children in community X is shown in the following list:

age (years)	male	female
0	23	17
1	23	19
2	21	17
3	18	16
4	14	12
5	13	12
6	13	15
7	14	14
8	14	15
9	12	13
10	13	14
11	12	14
12	12	13
13	11	13
14	10	11

(a)   Make three age groups (on the pattern of the census table at the beginning of the exercises).

(b)   What is the age and sex make-up in each group?

(c)   What percentage of the total population does each group constitute?

(d)   Draw a pie chart showing the three groups of children as segments of the total population.

APPENDICES

APPENDICES

Index to Appendices

To be copied for all participants

Appendix A.1   Pictures of Part A to be cut out

Appendix A.2   Possible solutions to exercises of Part A

Appendix A.3   Teaching games and questions bank

Appendix A.4   Problem tree and tree of objectives

Appendix B.1   Analysing health systems by means of indicators

                                        A.   What is an indicator
                                        B.   Indicators for a district health system
                                        C.   Additional indicators

Appendix B.2   Possible solutions to exercises Part B

Appendix B.3   Teaching games and questions bank

Appendix B.4   Statistical data

Appendix B.5   Exercise on the use of indicators

APPENDIX A.1
PICTURES OF PART A

(to be cut out)

1 Consultation book

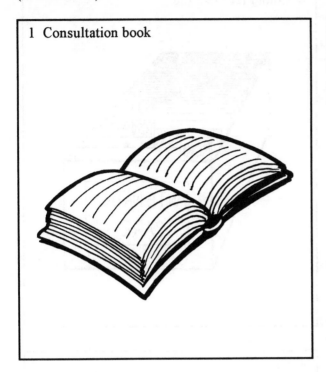

2 Annual report

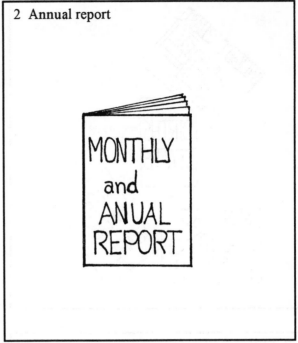

3 Chats with the community

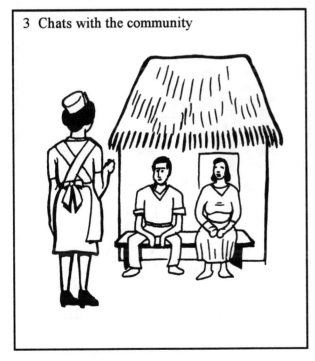

4 Cemetery

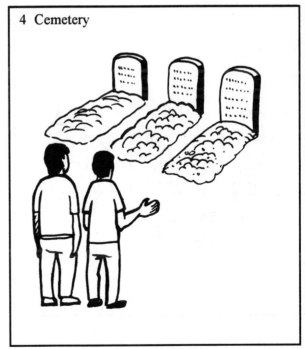

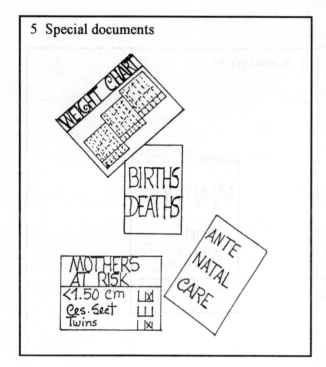

5 Special documents

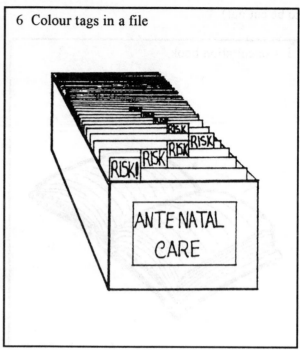

6 Colour tags in a file

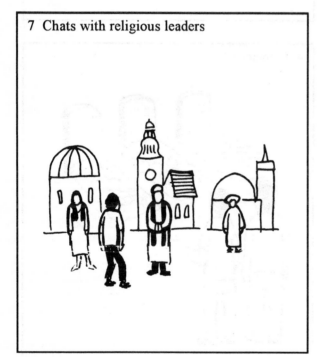

7 Chats with religious leaders

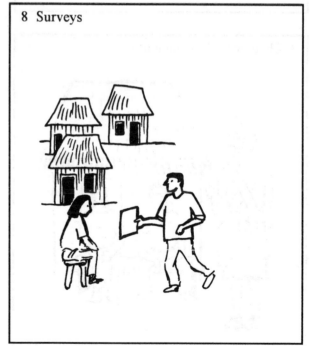

8 Surveys

9 Community A

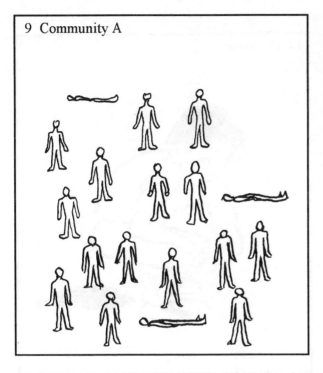

10 Community B

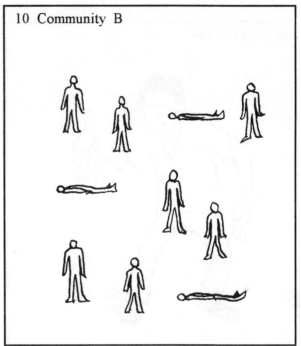

11 Accidents

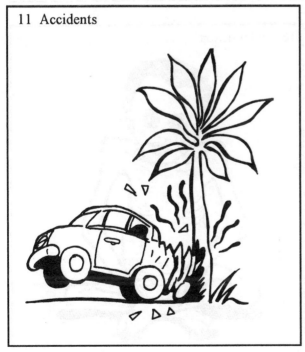

12 Mosquito reproduction (malaria)

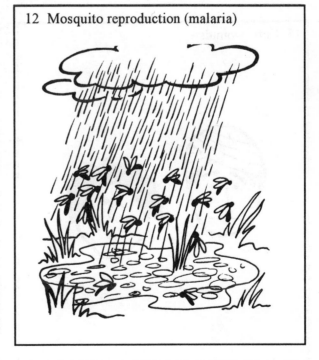

13 Drunkenness

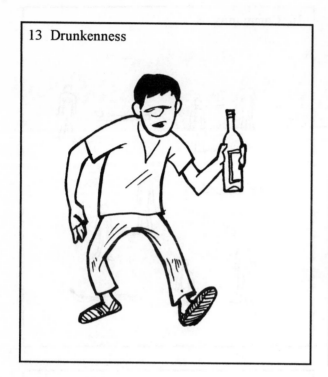

14 Diarrhoea

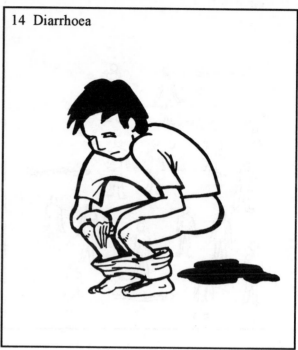

15 Cuts, wounds

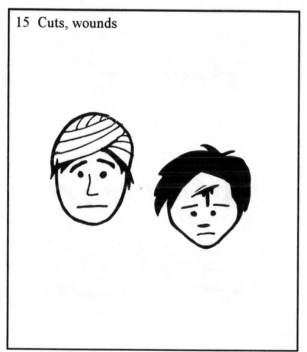

16 Malnutrition

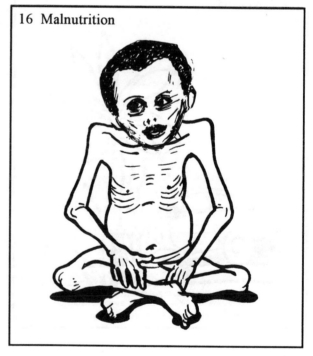

17 Epilepsy

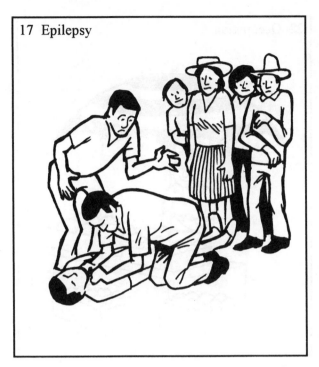

18 Tuberculosis

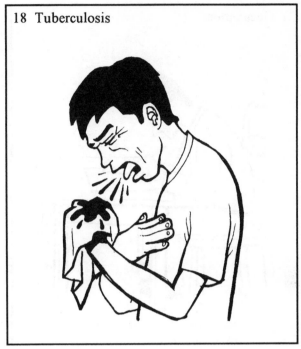

19 Occupation

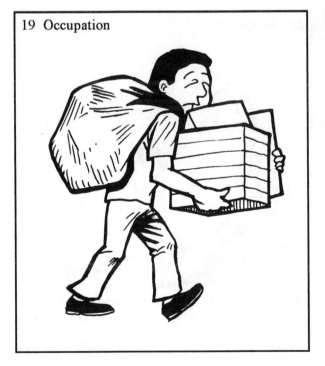

20 Occupation

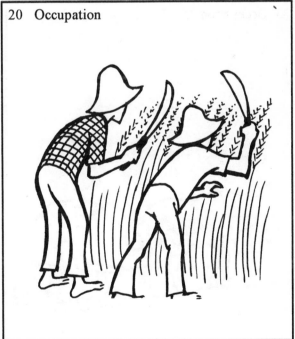

21 Occupation

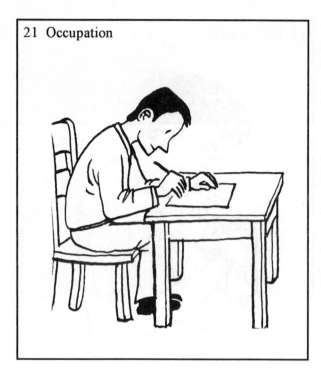

22 Occupation

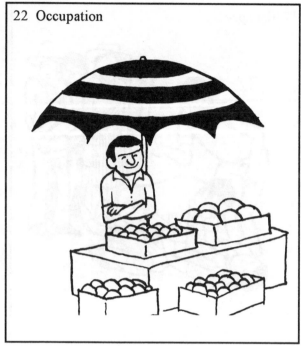

23 Occupation

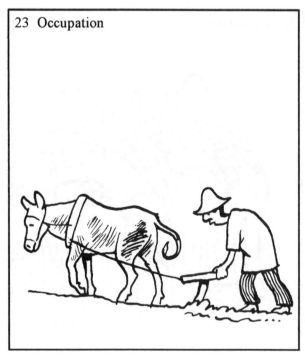

24 Occupation

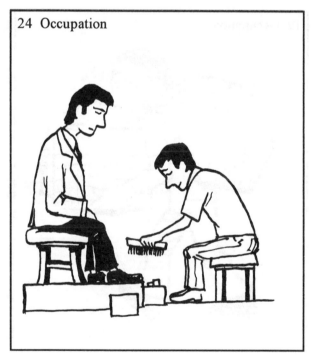

25 Literacy/Illiteracy

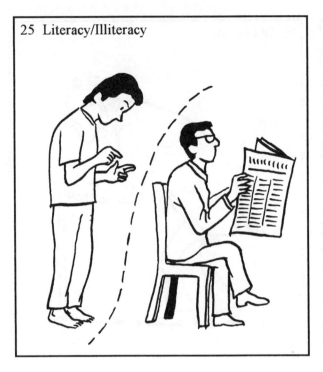

26 Distance to Health Posts

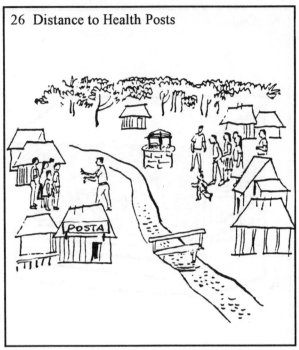

27 Under-fives

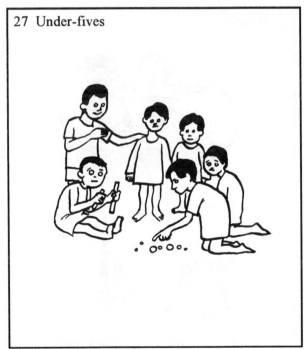

28 Schoolchildren

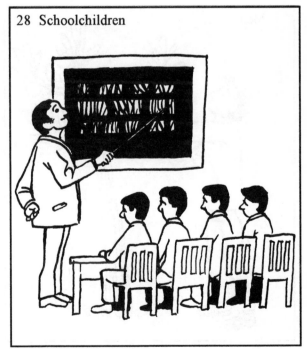

29 Adults

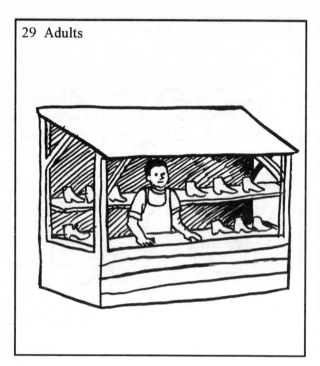

30 Old people

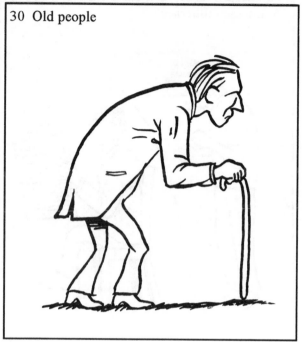

31 Men

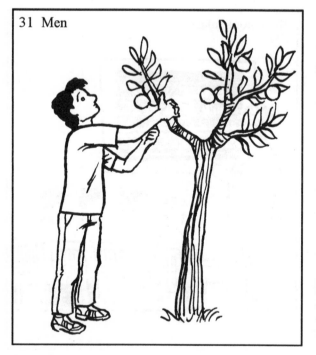

32 Women

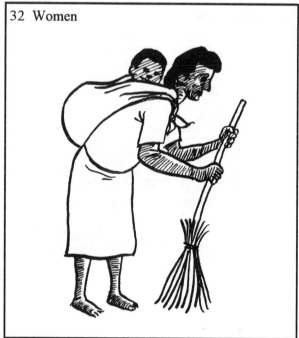

33 Rich people

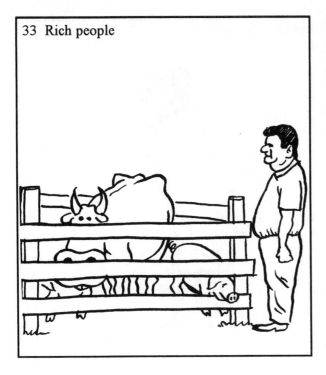

34 Poor people

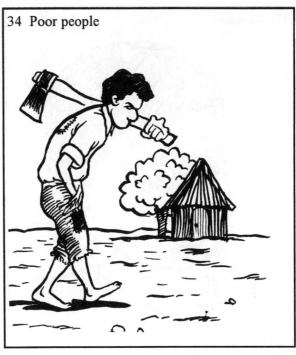

35 Wounds

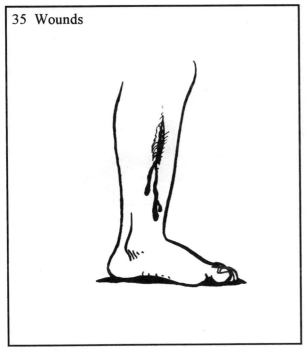

36 Burns

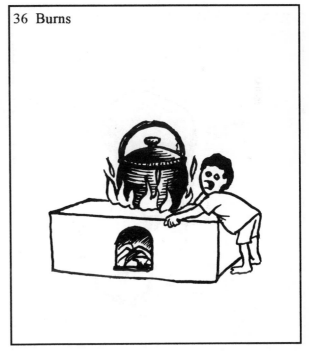

37 Measles

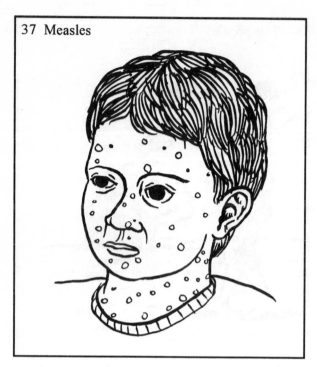

38 Back pain

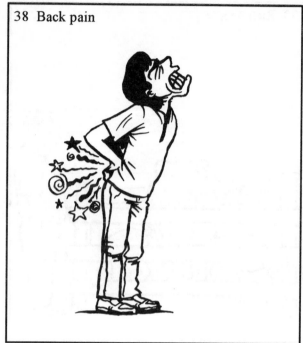

39 Malnutrition

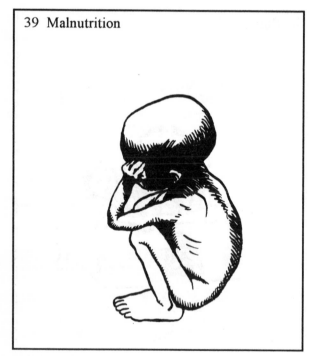

40 Alcoholism

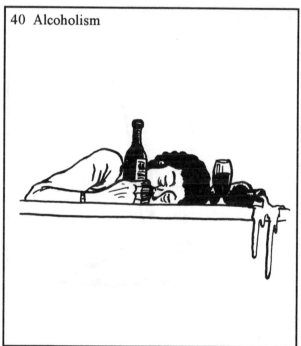

41 Problems in childbirth

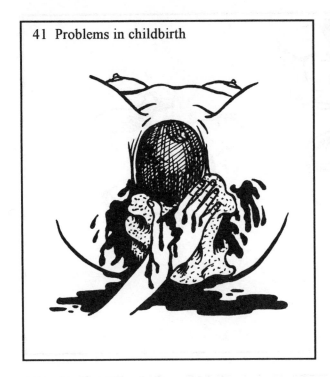

42 Obesity

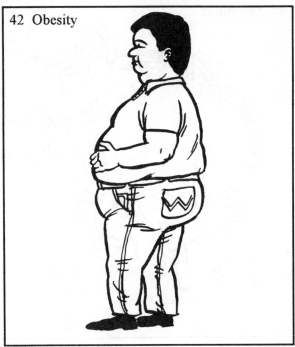

43 Treatments

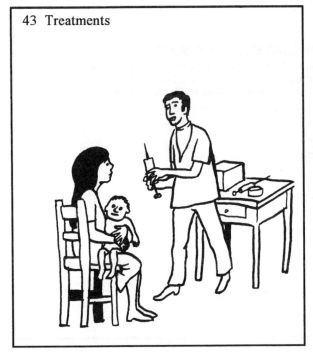

44 Rehabilitation

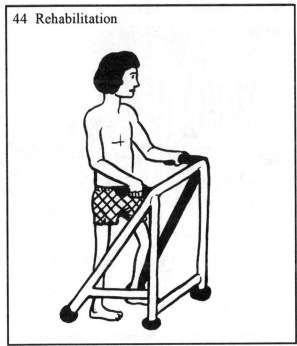

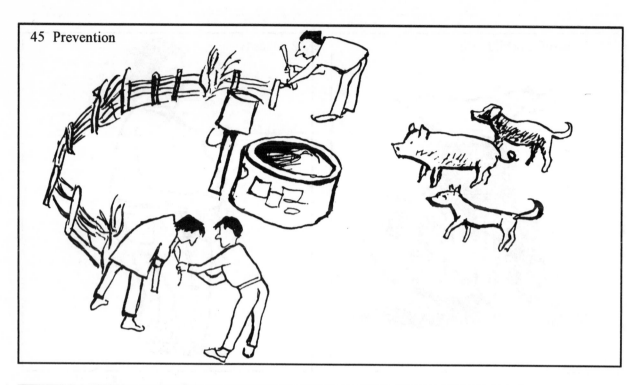

45 Prevention

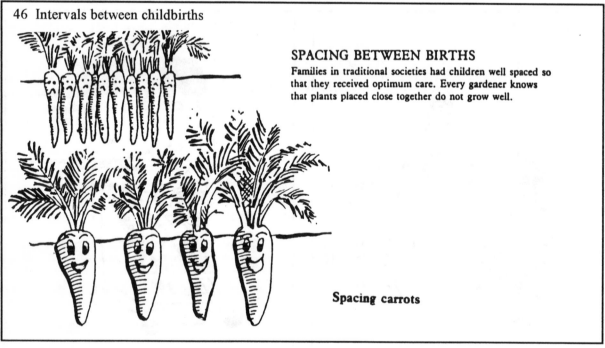

46 Intervals between childbirths

SPACING BETWEEN BIRTHS

Families in traditional societies had children well spaced so that they received optimum care. Every gardener knows that plants placed close together do not grow well.

Spacing carrots

47 Space between births

Spacing births reduces deaths

Bangladesh: World Fertility Survey

Spacing between births	Infant deaths/ 1000 births	Toddler deaths/ 1000 alive	Child deaths/ 1000 alive
	0-1st birthday	1st-2nd birthday	2nd-4th birthday
Less than 2 years	185	42	81
2-4 years	89	28	62
Over 4 years	58	10	27

All twenty-nine other countries studied showed similar trends

48 Infant mortality

Too young: Children born to women under the age of 20 are approximately twice as likely to die in infancy as children born to women in their mid-20s.

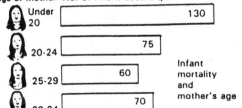

Age of mother — No. of infant deaths (per 1000 live births)

- Under 20: 130
- 20-24: 75
- 25-29: 60
- 30-34: 70

Infant mortality and mother's age

From a survey in Argentina

Too many: The risks to the health of both mother and infant increase steeply after the third child.

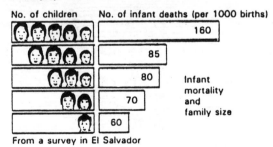

No. of children — No. of infant deaths (per 1000 births)

- 160
- 85
- 80
- 70
- 60

Infant mortality and family size

From a survey in El Salvador

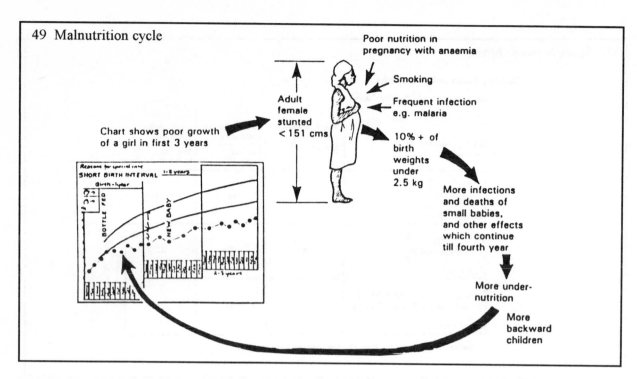

49 Malnutrition cycle

Poor nutrition in pregnancy with anaemia

Smoking

Frequent infection e.g. malaria

Chart shows poor growth of a girl in first 3 years

Adult female stunted < 151 cms

10% + of birth weights under 2.5 kg

More infections and deaths of small babies, and other effects which continue till fourth year

More under-nutrition

More backward children

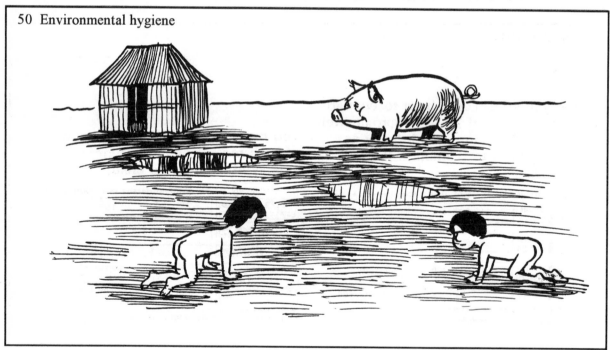

50 Environmental hygiene

51 Birth with severe problems

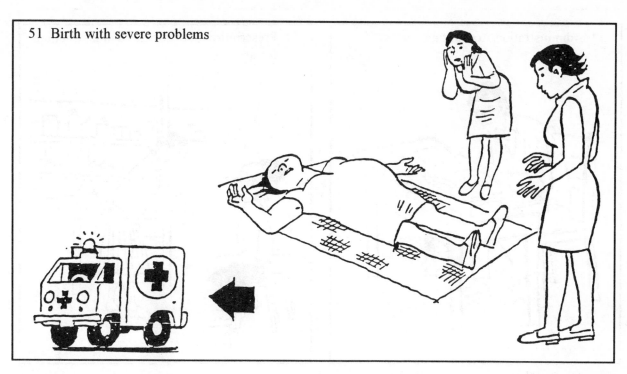

52 Risk factors at birth

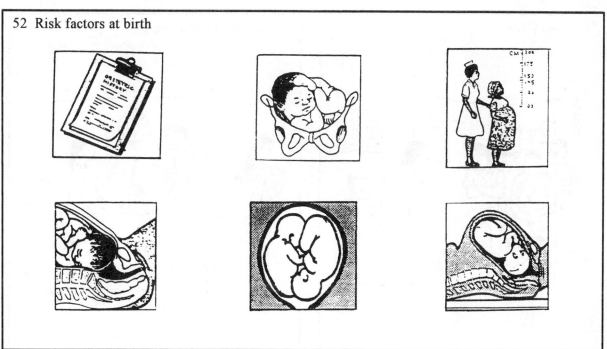

53 Administration/Accounting

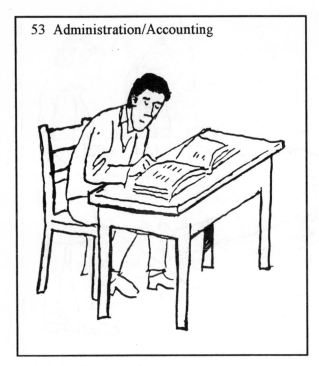

54 Prescription of medicines and instructions for use

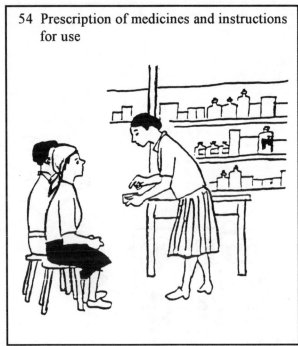

55 Home visits

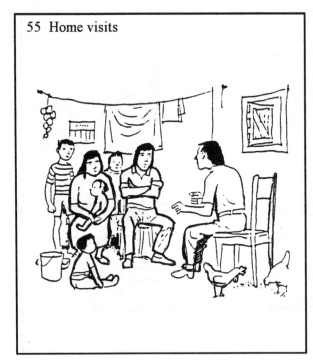

56 Growth monitoring

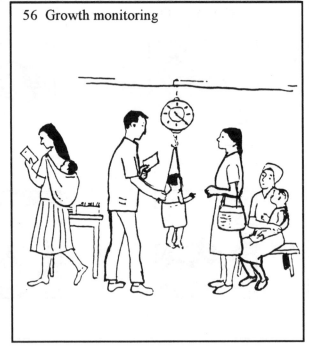

57 Community meetings

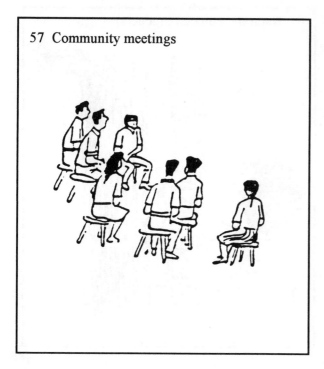

58 Examination of sputum (TBC)

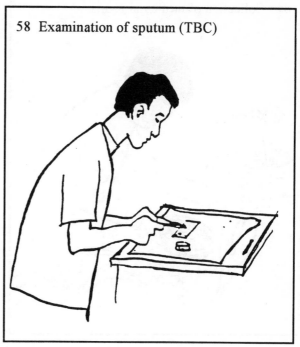

59 Stool examinations

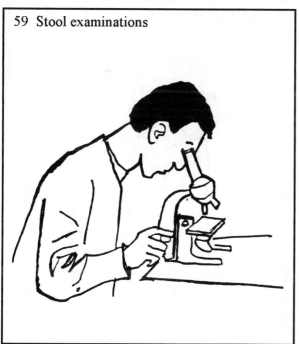

60 Health education for TB patients

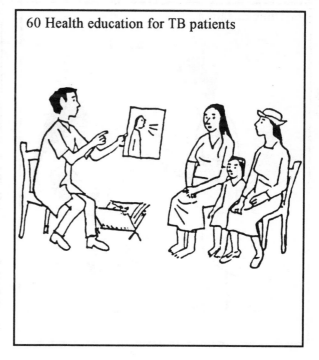

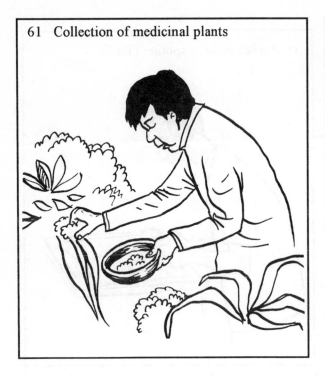

61 Collection of medicinal plants

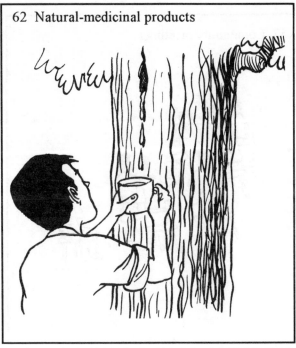

62 Natural-medicinal products

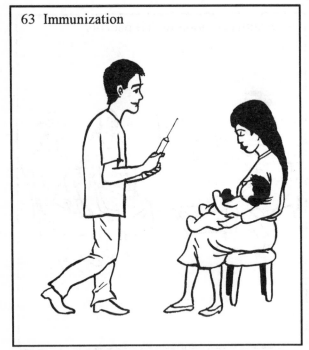

63 Immunization

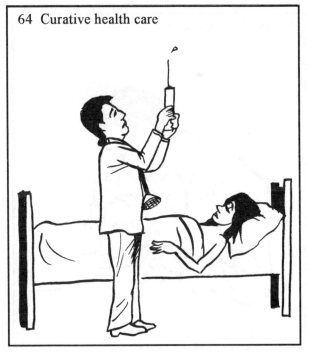

64 Curative health care

65 Rehabilitation

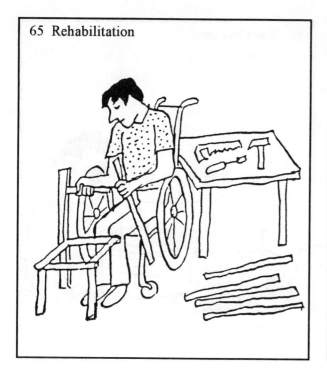

66 Water supply

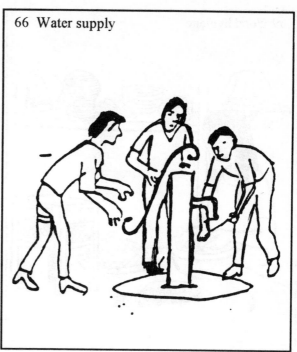

67 Nutrition

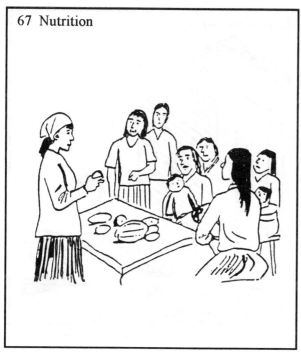

68 Breast feeding

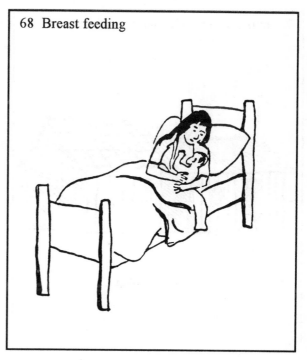

69 Food hygiene

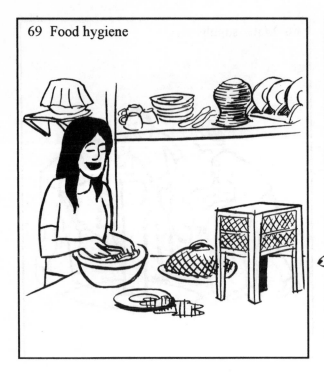

70 Water hygiene

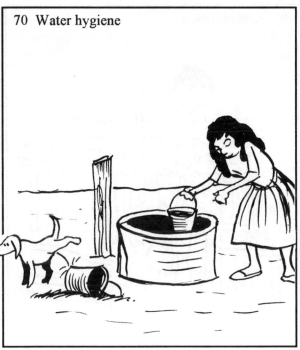

71 Improvement of housing

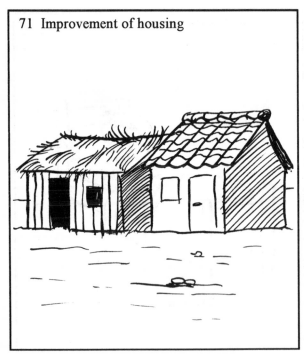

72 Improve latrines

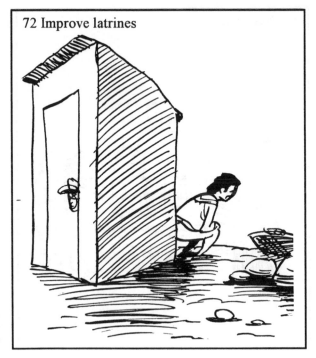

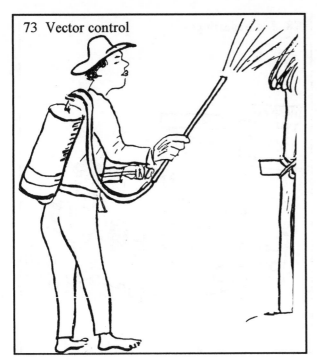

73 Vector control

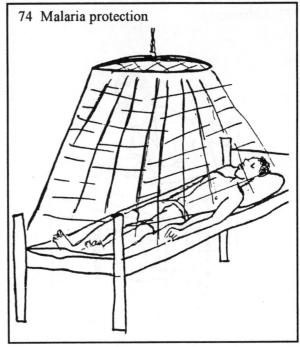

74 Malaria protection

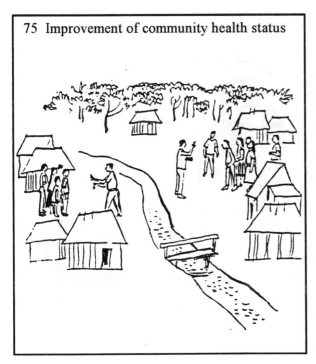

75 Improvement of community health status

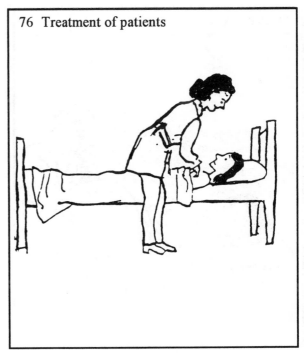

76 Treatment of patients

77 Statistics

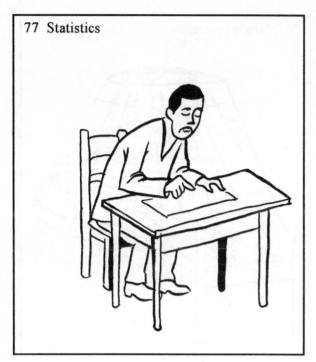

78 Team meetings

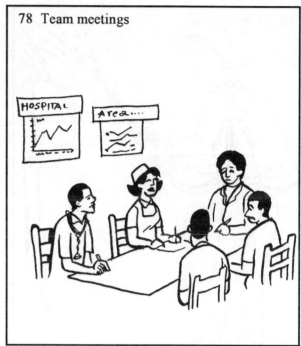

79 Delivery

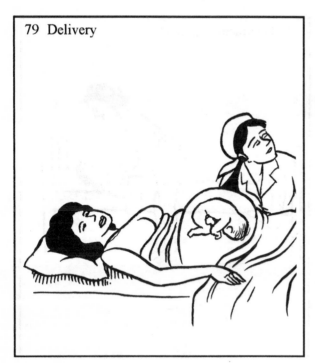

80 Antenatal control

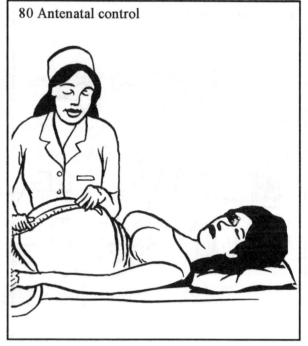

81
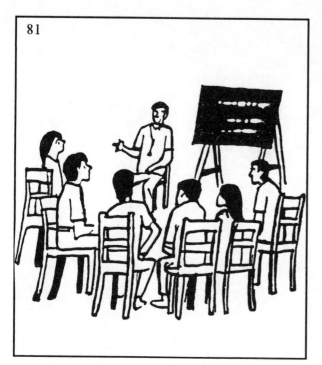

82
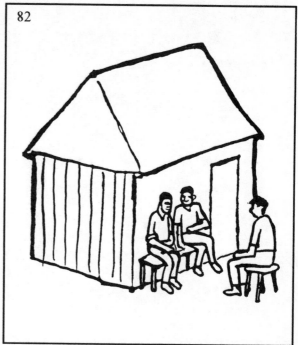

83
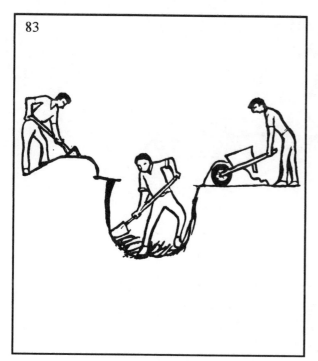

84
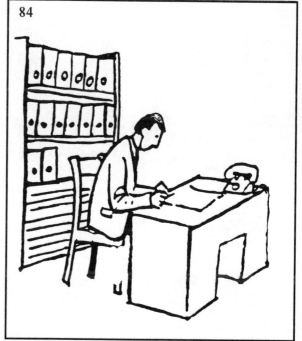

APPENDIX A.2

POSSIBLE SOLUTIONS TO EXERCISES IN PART A

Page 25   **Proportions and graphical representation**

(a)   Community B is healthier than Community A because more of its members are healthy per total population.

(b)   Proportion = Comparative relationship of parts in a whole

Proportion allows the comparison of the frequency or magnitude of events in different populations or population groups. For instance, the proportion of sick people in a community is calculated by dividing the number of sick persons (in the whole population or in a specific age group) by the total number of people (sick and healthy in the whole population or in a specific age group). The proportion is frequently expressed as a percentage (%). (Note: prepare a special evening session for those participants who do not know how to calculate percentages).

A similar concept is that of *rate*. *The mortality* or *morbidity rate* is the number of persons dying or falling ill within a given period of time divided by the total number of persons observed.

(c)   Graphical representation: proportions expressed in four pie charts.

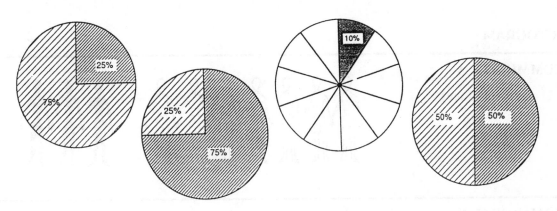

Two additional pie charts.

Community A

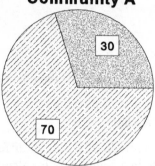

Community B

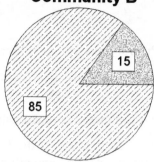

3 out of ten are sick (30%)

$$\frac{3}{10} \times 100$$

3 out of twenty are sick (15%)

$$\frac{3}{20} \times 100$$

(d)   Expressing proportions in pictograms

PICTOGRAM

COMMUNITY A (3 out of ten)	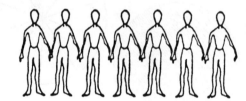 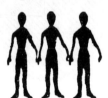
COMMUNITY B (1.5 out of ten)	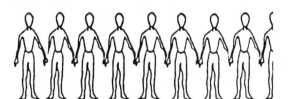 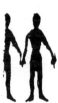

Page 28 **Graphical representation for seasonal variations**

Some health events are more likely to occur :

●   at a particular time of the year (seasonal): malaria, diarrhoea, cuts (at harvest time), malnutrition

●   during the weekend: drunkenness, cuts (due to violence), accidents

●   working days: traffic accidents (during rush hours), cuts (incurred at home or in the work-place, resulting from violence).

Other health events like tuberculosis, epilepsy and chronic diseases are not time-or season-related events, they occur throughout the year.

Page 29 **Graphical representation for seasonal variations (2nd example)**

Questions a, b, and c Admissions to hospital because of diarrhoea and cholera, per month

Questions d and e During the rainy season, flooding may spread refuse and faecal matter over large areas, contaminating wells in the process. In other areas, diarrhoeal diseases occur more frequently during the dry season. This is due to the fact that the few wells that do not dry up do not suffice to meet the needs of both humans and livestock

       Well preservation and other water-conservation measures should be taken to provide the population with clean drinking water all year round.

Page 29 **Drawing a sketch map or a diagram**

This could prove useful for the planning of health interventions (discuss examples of this).

The following pictures represent simple and sophisticated versions of the problem to be solved:

(a) Simple version

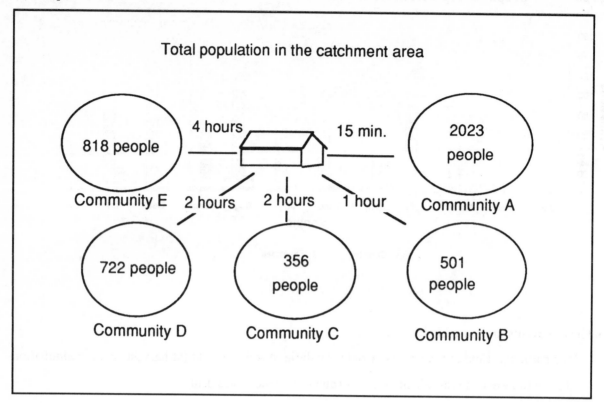

Total population in the catchment area

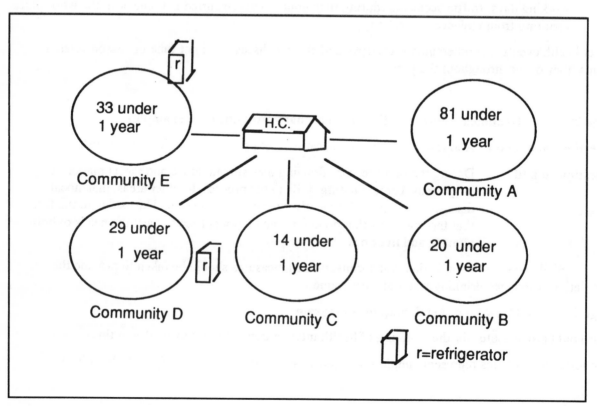

(b) Two more sophisticated versions

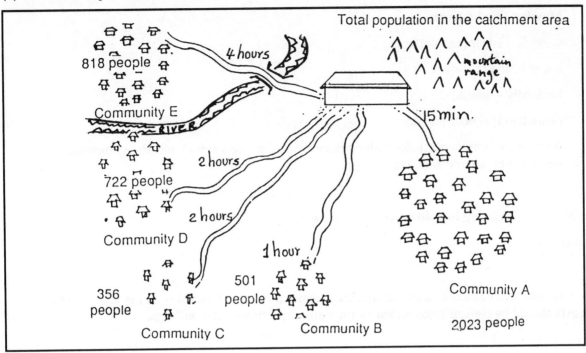

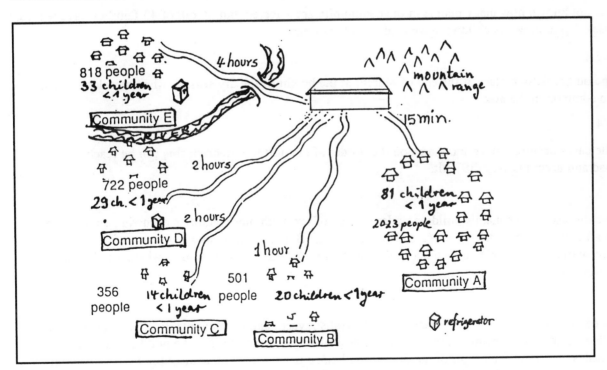

Page 32   **Risk groups**

(a)   Measles – under-fives;

wounds – sugar cane cutters;

burns – small children;

back pain – adults;

malnutrition – poor people.

(b)   Analysis of documents, talks with community leaders, community meetings, surveys, participants' observation, etc.

Page 39   **Training in epidemiological thinking**

Answers to

Q.1

There has been an outbreak of a communicable disease, presumably measles, in the village. The diagnosis should be clinically confirmed by the nurse reporting on the outbreak.

Q.2

It is not known how many people in the community are affected, but 30 out of 45 families have reported cases. Up to now, six children have died from the disease.

Q.3

The outbreak took place at the end of March, at the height of the dry season, when measles epidemics are common in the area.

Q.4

The cases occurred in a remote area on the border of the northern district; this can be reached only by road and access is very difficult.

Q.5

The disease affects mainly children under the age of six, with most fatalities occurring among very small children (less than three years old) and infants. But some adolescents are also affected. No information is available on whether the outbreak struck families at random or whether risk factors played a role.

Q.6

Since measles epidemics have occurred in the last six years and no immunization team has visited the village in at least as many years, immunity has probably been lowered to the point that exposure to measles viruses at the height of the dry season helped trigger this epidemic outbreak. The general condition of those affected seems to lend some weight to this theory, but information on the immunization status of the community (Cf. Q.5) should be sought to confirm it.

Q.7

The headman of the village ordered a sort of quarantine in order to reduce contacts. But the villagers, who make witchcraft responsible for the epidemic, do not seek help at the dispensary in G.

Q.8

The spread of the disease has not yet ended and six infants have already died. Further information about the allegations of witchcraft (has anyone been singled out?) may prove useful when conducting an information campaign on the actual causes of the disease.

Q.9

A mobile team could be sent to the village in order to give symptomatic treatment to the diseased children and to detect infants at risk of dying, who should then be treated to prevent complications. There is no need to immunize children in the stricken village itself (because most of them are already infected), but completion of measles immunization in nearby villages, where no vaccination has taken place in the last three years, should be considered. It is doubtful whether the imposition of some sort of quarantine could be of any use in this situation. An information campaign on the causes of measles should be carried out for social reasons.

Page 42   Risk factors

Show picture 52 as answer to 4b

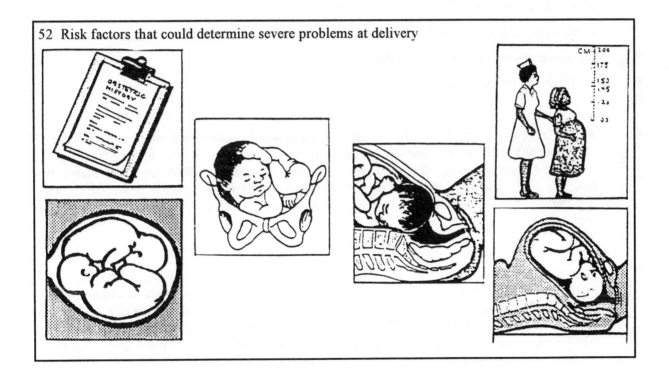

52 Risk factors that could determine severe problems at delivery

Page 44   An epidemic outbreak

1. A cholera outbreak is suspected. The village should be closely supervised starting with the first field visit, as the clinical picture, with absence of fever, high case-fatality rate and dehydration followed by coma, suggests the possibility of a cholera outbreak.

2. You should conduct a household survey during the course of this epidemic outbreak to collect all possible data on morbidity and mortality.

- Screening of all villagers should take place to detect all unreported cases.

- All possible water sources used by the village population should be identified, inspected and chlorinated.

- You should inform yourself about the general sanitary picture of the village (waste disposal and the like).

3. The situation calls for immediate action in order to avoid further propagation of the disease and a higher death toll:

- Inform the villagers of the nature of the disease and tell them what they should do

- Create a rehydration centre for intravenous and oral therapy

- Curb the number of public gatherings and outdoor events, or ban them altogether

- Impose an environmental cleaning campaign

- Control drinking water and food hygiene

- Recommend construction and use of latrines

- Verify diagnosis by bacteriological means.

4. Since a large number of those infected with the bacterium do not develop the disease (iceberg phenomenon), chemoprophylaxis as well as post-exposure immunization is no longer considered essential. As to ORT, when applied early it can considerably reduce case-fatality. In this case, too, it appears that the decrease in disease transmission followed a natural course and that the day it set in just happened to coincide with that on which chemoprophylaxis was initiated.

5. Whereas for classical cholera 59% of those infected remain symptom-free and the disease manifests itself in severe form in only 11% of all cases, for the El Tor cholera, the figures are 75% and 2%, respectively. Generally speaking, only 20 to 50 per cent of the given population is likely to become infected with the El Tor strain. Thus, in a village with a total population of 1700, a maximum of 850 inhabitants are susceptible to the bacterium. Of these, only 17 (two per cent) are expected to be severe cases.

    A mere 22 cases were reported here (Fig. 2), and it appears most likely that the epidemic was about to run its natural course anyway.

APPENDIX A.3

DIDACTIC GAMES AND QUESTIONS BANK

FIRST DIDACTIC GAME: THE SNAIL

Plan (board)

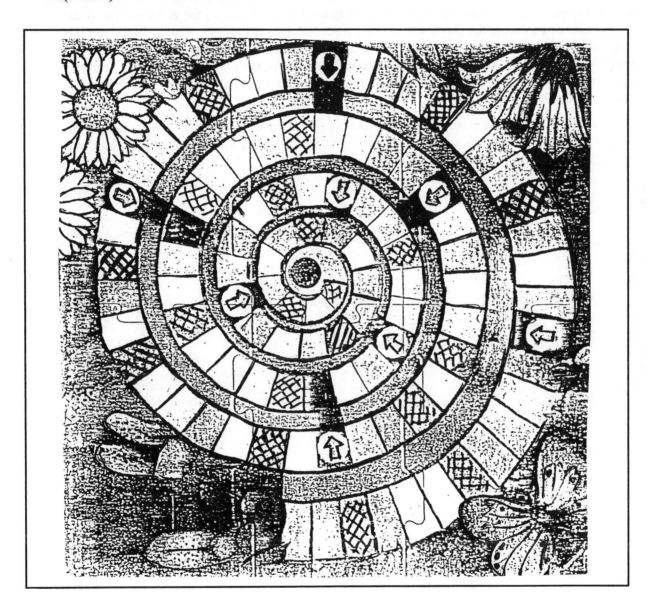

Rules

Each player is given one pawn. If more than six players are to take part in the game, teams of two each should be formed.

Each player throws the dice and moves his/her pawn as many squares ahead as determined by the final roll of the dice (one, two, three, four, five or six squares for as many spots on the side of the dice that is facing upward).

Should the pawn land on a shaded square, the player must draw one card from the stack and answer the question on it, the other players deciding on the correctness of the given answer. If the answer is deemed wrong, the player has to move back one, two or three squares. If the answer is considered correct, the player can stay on the shaded square until his/her turn to throw the dice comes again. When the pawn lands on a square marked with an arrow, the player must draw one card from the stack and answer the question on it. If this answer is regarded as correct by the other participants, the player can move to the next square.

The facilitator can clarify questions whenever the need arises and can even add sub questions. To win this game, a player must come as close as possible to the centre of the board and get there first, or lead the field after a predetermined time has elapsed.

Questions Bank

Name four epidemiological questions which refer to the magnitude and distribution of a health problem or health event.	Which epidemiological questions refer to action to be taken? (Name three)
Provide two examples showing the usefulness of the epidemiological questions in your own work.	How can you represent results on 'where did a particular event occur?'
In your opinion, what is a population?	How do you define 'magnitude' of diarrhoeal diseases?
State three direct and three indirect causes of diarrhoeal diseases in a community	What are some of the difficulties of supervising lower-level health personnel?
You have just performed an intervention to alleviate a health problem What should be your next step?	What is epidemiology? (Give a rough definition).
What does the following question mean: 'Where do the cases occur?'	In your opinion, what is a community?
Name three of the advantages of dealing with health problems in communities (instead of only in individuals)	What is the first of the Nine Epidemiological Questions?
What purpose do the Nine Epidemiological Questions serve?	

SECOND DIDACTIC GAME. 'COMING FULL CIRCLE'

Plan

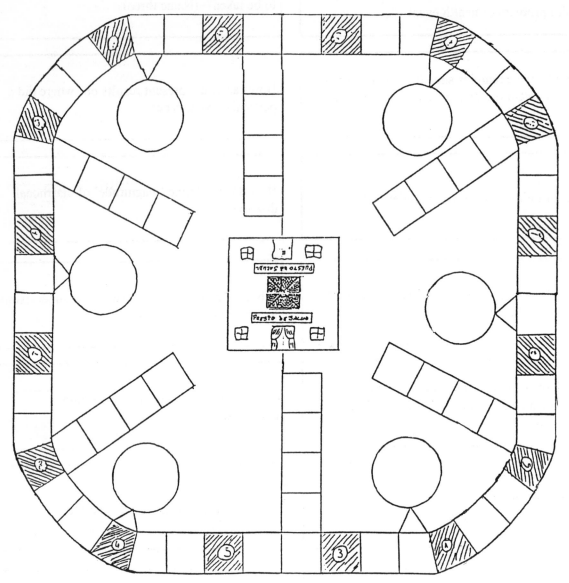

Rules

The object of this game is for the players to complete as rapidly as possible the entire circle-like course, exiting through the 'gate' closest to their respective starting point. The rules are those of the Snail Game, except that players giving the wrong answer to the question drawn are required to move back four positions. Besides, a pawn is to be moved back to its previous position on the board if others catch up with it, for no more than one pawn at a time can occupy the same position. This, however, does not apply to the so-called 'squares of peace,' (represented by the shaded squares) where two or more pawns may stand together at any one time.

The second set of questions covers the first two epidemiological questions.

Questions Bank

How can we measure health status? (Give four examples).	In a community of 600 inhabitants, ten per cent suffer from persistent coughing. How many persons have this condition?
Three out of ten in a community are ill. Express this as a percentage.	What does 'mortality rate' in a community mean?
What is 'health status' in a community?	In community A, ten persons have tuberculosis and in community B, only five. Which of the two communities is more affected by tuberculosis?
Draw a pictogram to show that three out of ten children have had diarrhoea.	What does 'morbidity rate' in a community mean?
Name three health problems that are likely to respond to public health measures?	During a community meeting, how would you go about getting information on people's health problems?
A health problem is susceptible to public health measures. Explain this.	Name three health problems that are unlikely to respond to public health measures
For what purposes can you use colour tags in a file?	What are the main disadvantages of a health survey?

Name four criteria (or characteristics) of a health problem that show you that it is a very important one.

What is a percentage?

Twenty-four per cent of the population is currently suffering from a cold. Show this in a pie chart.

How can you assess the severity of a disease?

Children make up 45 per cent of the population of a given community. Show this in a pie chart.

How can you assess whether a health problem requires priority action?

THIRD DIDACTIC GAME: CIRCLES (all the way)

Plan

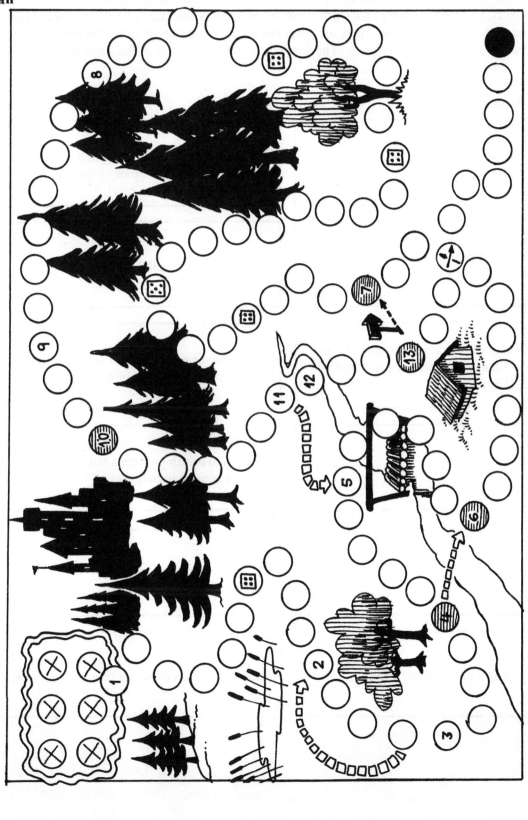

Rules

Each player receives one token. If there are more than six players, groups of two can be formed. Each player throws the dice and moves his token forward so many places (circles) as the number indicated by the position taken for the dice. The rules are as follows: if the player reaches a shaded (or numbered) circle, the player has to take a card from the question bank and answer the question written on it. If the answer is correct, he goes four places forward; if not, he remains in the same place. Two tokens can occupy the same position on a circle. There are other circles numbered which order the player to go forward or back a given number of places. The first to reach the last circle of the game wins.

Questions Bank

Name two health problems that occur at a particular time of the week	How can you represent in a graph the diseases occurring at different times of the year?
Do you think that maps are useful in your work? What for?	What is a linear graph?
You have a map of the catchment area of your health unit. What information items would you draw on it? (Give four).	Name three occupations that entail particular risks of contracting certain diseases
What is a 'risk group?'	Name three health problems not subject to marked seasonal variations
What is a 'risk factor'?	Where can you find information about risk groups in a population?
What does 'seasonal variation' mean?	Name some indirect causes of a health problem?

What is meant by 'coverage?'	How can you identify particular risk groups in a population?
What is the risk approach useful for?	For what purposes is the 'causation tree' useful?
Name three health problems which occur at particular times of the year.	What data can you collect on the activities of health personnel?

APPENDIX A.4

CAUSATION TREE (SIMPLIFIED)

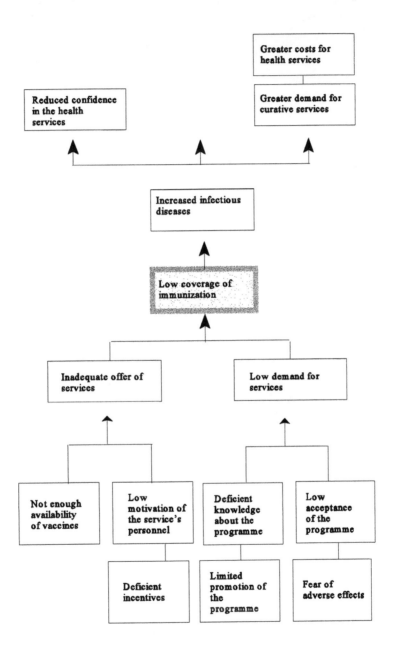

CAUSATION TREE (SIMPLIFIED)

APPENDIX B.1
ASSESSING DISTRICT HEALTH SYSTEMS
BY MEANS OF INDICATORS

A. WHAT IS AN INDICATOR?

Indicators are a measure that can be used to help describe a situation that exists and to measure changes or trends over a period of time. Most health indicators are quantitative in nature, but some are more qualitative.

The District Health Management Team needs to use health indicators to analyse the district's commitment to policies for socio-economic development and PHC (Primary Health Care), to monitor progress in implementing health programmes, and to evaluate their impact on the health status of the population. Health indicators are necessary in order to:

- Analyse the present situation.
- Make comparisons.
- measure changes over time (Vaughan, Morrow 1989).

So an indicator is a measurable characteristic or variable.

If you have to measure complex variables – such as social class, accessibility of health services, malnutrition, attitudes towards health services – you have to analyse the different dimensions of the variable and search for indicators that are able to measure them.

The *validity of an indicator* refers to the degree to which an indicator measures what it is designed to measure. The concept of validity includes measures of *sensitivity* and *specificity*.

For instance, the infant mortality rate (IMR) is a direct measure of the mortality of infants in their first year of life and it is at the same time an indirect measure of the health situation of a given population and of its overall socio-economic development. So it is a sensitive indicator of the infants' risk of dying but it is an unspecific indicator of the results of the health services' efforts because the reduction of IMR is influenced by many different socio-economic factors.

However useful an indicator may be, there are technical and financial problems in collecting the necessary data. But how accurate and valid does the data have to be for the indicator to be useful? This varies with the indicator and how it is going to be used. For analysing the present situation and for making rough comparisons, indicators for use in policy-making and health programme management do not need to be highly accurate. For instance, it is usually sufficient to know that the IMR is between 40 and 60 per 1000 or 100 and 120 per 1000, or over 150 per 1000.

However, when *measuring changes* in health status over relatively short periods of time, such as five years, much greater accuracy is required. For instance, the IMR needs to be carefully calculated if it is to be used as a measure of the improvement in the district's health status. In these situations, a trend over some time is the best indication that the situation is either improving, deteriorating or remains unchanged (Vaughan, Morrow 1989).

Although it is desirable to use quantitative indicators, it has to be taken into account that they describe only selected aspects of reality (i.e. of a complex variable). In some cases the qualitative description of the

131

phenomena observed reflects reality much better than quantitative indicators; i.e. the communication within the health team or between staff and communities. Frequently, both quantitative and qualitative (descriptive) approaches complement each other.

Quantitative indicators are expressed by numbers and percentages.

Qualitative indicators are descriptive. (Some authors do not use the term indicator for the 'qualitative' – i.e. non-numerical – description of the reality).

Example for the operationalization of a complex variable. (Canales et al, 1986)

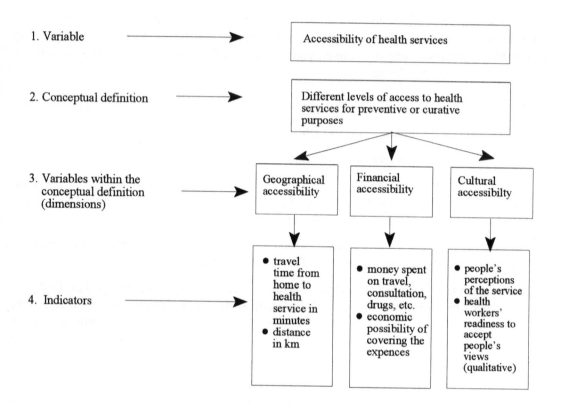

B.   INDICATORS FOR DISTRICT HEALTH SYSTEMS

(Main source: Pabón 1985 modified)

Conceptual framework for the evaluation of health services

Input*	1. Accessibility
	2. Availability

Process	3. Activities**
	4. Productivity
	5. Use
	6. Utilization
	7. Quality

Output (direct results)	8. Coverage
	9. Efficiency
	10. Efficacy

Outcome (impact on population)	11. Effectiveness

*   Sometimes called 'structure indicators.'

**   Activities may be interpreted as an input and/or as the result of the health services efforts. However, in this framework it is seen as an indicator which measures merely what is happening within the health services.

Input indicators

1.   Accessibility

The extent to which the population in need can use the service.

Examples:

Problem areas	Indicators
Geographical accessibility	distance travel time (according to transport media)
Economic accessibility	fees for services, drugs, travel expenditure (in relation to wages)
Cultural accessibility	acceptance of health services by people from other ethnic groups (qualitative); no. of rejections of people from different ethnic groups
Accessibility regarding organizational issues	waiting time; no. of rejections

2.   Availability

The ratio between existing resources and population.

Examples:

$$\frac{\text{No. of VHW*}}{\text{reference population}}$$

$$\frac{\text{No. of physicians*}}{\text{reference population}} \qquad \frac{\text{No. of health centres}}{\text{reference population}}$$

Process indicators

3.   Activities

The human and physical resources have to fulfil certain functions in order to reach their objectives. These functions are measured in terms of activities.

Examples:

Resources	Indicators (related to time)
Vaccination equipment	no. of doses vaccinated (according to vaccine, 1st, 2nd, 3rd, dose)
Ante-natal care unit	no. of pregnant women in ante-natal care,
Outpatient clinic	no. of consultations (according to type, speciality, etc.)

Time per activity (variable according to health unit and type of staff)

growth/assessment	10 minutes
ante-natal care	15 minutes
consultation	15 minutes
community visits	360 minutes
birth attendance	240 minutes
family planning	10 minutes
TB control (cases under treatment)	15 minutes

---

*   It is preferable to use the monthly or annual working hours

4.   Productivity and yield

The ratio between number of activities and time available per resource.

Examples:

$$\frac{\text{No. of antenatal controls}}{\text{no. of working hours of VHW*}}$$

$$\frac{\text{No. of growth assessments}}{\text{no. of working hours of VHW}}$$

If one allocates to each specific activity an expected average time, it is possible to calculate the productivity of any health worker by dividing the time used for specific activities by the number of hours hired.

Example:

$$\frac{(\text{No. of antenatal controls per year} \times 15) + (\text{N}^{\text{o}}. \text{ of consultations} \times 15) + ...}{\text{total working minutes contracted per year}}$$

Yield is different from productivity because the denominator is 'hours actually worked' instead of 'working hours hired'. However, generally it is very difficult to get information about 'hours actually worked'.

Example:

$$\frac{\text{No. of consultations}}{\text{hours worked in practice}}$$

---

*   VHW (Village Health Workers)
'working hours' = 'the hired hours'

5.   Use

5.1   The **intensity of use** (or concentration) is the average number of services (e.g. ante-natal care) users have received during a time period.

Indicators: ratio between number of activities received and number of users.

Service	Indicators (period = 1 year)
Outpatient clinic	no. of consultations
	no of outpatients*
Ante-natal care	no. of ante-natal controls
	no. of pregnant women attending
TBC-control	no. of TBC consultations
	no. of patients with TBC

* new patients during the time period

5.2   **Extent of use** (user rate):   the proportion of a given population which actually uses a service in a time period.

Indicator: percentage of first time users (in a year) of the reference population

Example:

Service	Indicators (period = 1 year)
Health post	$\dfrac{\text{no. of users (first time)}}{\text{reference population}} \times 100$

Frequently it is impossible to get clean data about first time users. Therefore the figure 'number of consultations per person per year' is used, which is a blend of the intensity and extent of use of health services.

136

6. Utilization

Utilization is the relationship between the actual use and the availability of resources per time unit.

Examples:

Resource	Indicators
Outpatient clinic	no. of real working hours (e.g. nurses)
	no. of contracted working hours
Surgery	no. of hours theatre used
	no. of hours theatre available

Note: Hospital utilization can be measured by means of three indicators:

$$\% \text{ occupation} = \frac{\text{no. occupied bed days}}{\text{no. of available bed days}}$$

$$\text{average length of stay} = \frac{\text{no. of occupied bed days}}{\text{no. of discharges}}$$

$$\text{productivity} = \frac{\text{no. of discharges}}{\text{no. of beds}}$$

7. Quality

Quality is a combination of characteristics – human and technological – which health services must possess in order to reach their objectives.

There are four elements of quality:

(a) to satisfy the patients' needs

(b) to do all that has to be done (minimum standard of care)

(c) to have the necessary skills

(d) to work in an appropriate time sequence

Medical audit is one way of measuring quality. Patients' satisfaction with different aspects of the service can be measured by means of questionnaires.

Output indicators

8. Coverage

Coverage is the proportion of people with a need for health services who actually receive such services within a given time.

Examples:

Service	Indicators	
Vaccination	$\dfrac{\text{no of vaccinated target children}}{\text{no. of target children}}$	x 100
Ante-natal care	$\dfrac{\text{no. of target women with ante-natal care}}{\text{no. of target women}}$	x 100
Birth attendance	$\dfrac{\text{no. of attended births}}{\text{no. of expected births}}$	x 100
Outpatient clinic	$\dfrac{\text{no. of consultations}}{\text{no. of persons in need *}}$	x 100
Water supply	$\dfrac{\text{households with water supply}}{\text{no. of households}}$	x 100

* difficult to assess. Therefore, it is often impossible to calculate the coverage of curative services.

9. Efficacy

Efficacy refers to the objectives achieved by the service with respect to the individual user.

Examples:

Service	Indicators	
Immunization programme	$\dfrac{\text{no. of children effectively protected *}}{\text{no. of children vaccinated}}$	x 100
TB Control	$\dfrac{\text{no. of TB patients cured}}{\text{no. of TB patients treated}}$	x 100
Outpatient clinic	$\dfrac{\text{no. of patients cured}}{\text{no. of patients treated}}$	x 100

* According to the level of antibodies

10. Efficiency

Efficiency shows the relationship between the outputs of a programme or health service and the corresponding costs of the resources per time span.

Examples:

Service	Indicators	
Immunization programme	costs of the programme	
	no. of patients cured*	
TB control	costs of the TB programme	
	number of patients cured	
VHW (village health worker)	costs of the VHW programme	
	no. of activities	
Budget utilization (absorption capacity)	money spent for activities	x 100
	available budget	

* sometimes the number of patients attended is taken

11.   Effectiveness

Effectiveness is the result of health actions in the target population. (It is frequently impossible to distinguish whether any improvements in health are due to socio-economic development or arise directly from health service interventions.)

Examples:

Needs and strategies	Indicators
Multisectoral strategies	Improvement of birth rates, fertility rates, crude mortality rate, infant mortality rate
MCH programmes	Reduction of maternal mortality rate, percentage of low–birth–weight babies, malnutrition rate, prenatal, neonatal, infant mortality rate, incidence of EPI* target diseases
Malaria control TBC control	Reduction of malaria incidence Prevalence of TBC

*EPI = expanded programme of immunization

Effectiveness is sometimes calculated as the difference of rates between different years (also called 'effect' of health interventions) or as the percentage reduction over the years.

Example:

$$\frac{IMR^* \ 1985 - IMR \ 1990}{IMR \ 1985} \ x \ 100 \qquad\qquad \frac{95 - 85}{95} \ x \ 100 = 10.5\%$$

* IMR=Infant Mortality Rate

C. ADDITIONAL INDICATORS (GTZ/ITHÖG 1990. modified)

INPUT

Availability of standard equipment $=$ $\dfrac{\text{No. of health facilities with more than } x\% \text{ of equipment (according to list)}}{\text{total of health facilities}}$

A list of standard equipment for each type of health facility has to be worked out in advance. The indicator is a measure of the management's capacity to ensure the necessary continuous supply of essential equipment. The indicator can be applied to dispensable goods, such as drugs and vaccines.

PROCESS

Drop–out rate $=$ $\dfrac{\text{No. of patients not completing a treatment}}{\text{No. of patients beginning the treatment}}$ x 100

This indicator expresses the compliance with a long term treatment (e.g. TB or leprosy) or with a vaccination schedule (e.g. DPT, polio).

Functioning of the reporting system $=$ $\dfrac{\text{no. of reports available at a given time}}{\text{expected no. of reports}}$ x 100

The indicator does not measure the quality of information (except for including only complete or high standard reports) but only the quantity of reports. Furthermore, an indicator for the feedback to the primary level has to be considered.

Attendance rate of training courses $=$ $\dfrac{\text{no. of staff attending training courses}}{\text{total number of staff}}$ x 100

The indicator measures how training courses offered to different kinds of health personnel have been accepted. It does not measure the level of knowledge achieved.

Regularity of supervision $=$ $\dfrac{\text{no. of facilities supervised in the past } x \text{ months}}{\text{total number of health facilities}}$ x 100

The type of health facilities to be supervised, as well as the frequency, has to be determined in advance. If a standardized report is being used, the indicator provides an indirect estimate of the quality of supervising activities. One can also construct an additional indicator: number of complete filled reports/total number of reports.

Performance of
village health committees $=$ $\dfrac{\text{no. of meetings of village health committees in the past x months}}{\text{no. of meetings expected or planned}} \times 100$

This indicator does not measure the efficacy of village health committees or their impact on health but merely the number of meetings. However, these are a precondition for doing an effective job.

Knowledge/skills of staff $=$ $\dfrac{\text{no. of staff having x\% of standard knowledge/skill}}{\text{total number of staff}} \times 100$

Levels of standard knowledge for each category of staff have to be determined in advance and standardized tests have to be developed.

Budget utilization (absorption capacity) $=$ $\dfrac{\text{money spent on activities}}{\text{available budget}} \times 100$

APPENDIX B.2
POSSIBLE SOLUTIONS TO THE EXERCISES OF
PART B

Page 64   **Use of sketch maps**

Answer to:

(a)

Community	No. of consultations per person /semester	Proportion of patients with diarrhoea	Proportion of patients with malaria attacks
A	0.25	6%	16%
B	0.18	20%	16%
C	0.11	7%	15%
D	0.10	10%	31%
E	0.04	18%	12%

(b)

Diarrhoeal diseases seem to be more common both in community B and community E. It is very likely that the more severe cases are indigenous to community E, while less severe cases in the same community have most probably been brought in by visitors from distant communities.

As to community D, it has a particularly high proportion of people suffering from malaria attacks. This may be due to a greater predisposition of some community members to the disease, to a particularly marked tendency there of reporting fever cases as malaria, or to the presence of breeding-sites.

(c)

You could do a survey of all households or poll only some of them, asking about diarrhoeal diseases and malaria attacks in the two weeks preceding the interviews. This is not easy and should therefore be undertaken only with the help of the district health manager. (Description of the methods in: WHO 1988, Lutz 1986, Vaughan and Morrow 1989.)

(d) You can draw the following sketch and map

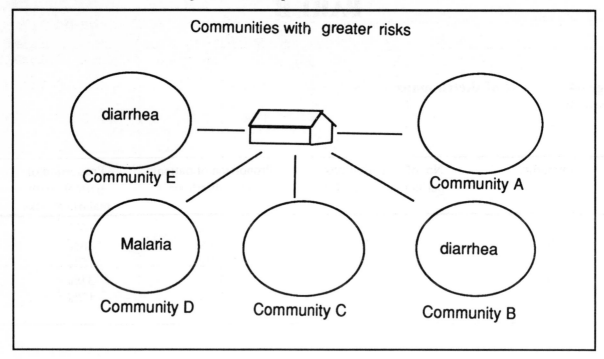

As an alternative, you can also draw pie charts on the map. You should visit the communities, analyse their specific characteristics (community diagnosis) and find explanations for the higher incidence of certain diseases there. This analysis must be seen as an essential step in controlling them.

Page 163   Indicators

1.   In order to be able to answer this question we would need a map and the information of travelling times (by car or boat) from each community to the central hospital. Then we would draw isocrones in our map, i.e. communities within 1 hour's travelling distance, 1 to 2 hours' travelling distance, etc. This allows us to estimate the proportion of the population (pregnant women) covered by emergency services.

2.   Availability of physicians   11/92500   =   0.1 per 1000
                        nurses   23/92500   =   0.2 per 1000
                        beds   77/92500   =   0.8 per 1000

3.   Main activities of physicians: outpatients
      nurses: preventive programmes, home visits

      Weak areas: birth attendance, vaccination

4.   Productivity (see table)

Type of activity	Total number of activities performed per year by		Total number of activities performed per day by		Minutes per day by	
	Physician	Midwives/ nurses	Physician	Midwives/ nurses	Physician	Midwives/ nurses
Consultations	15569	—	5.1	—	76.5	—
Weight monitoring	—	101	—	0.02	—	0.3
Birth attendance	250	729	0.08	0.11	9.6	26.4
Antenatal care	—	5257	—	—	—	4.15
Vaccination	250	292	0.08	0.83	0.4	3.75
Family planning	—	1584	—	0.25	—	7.65
Adult monitoring	—	3250	—	0.51	—	25.2
Home visits	—	1783	—	0.28	—	—
Total minutes					86.5	67.2
Total hours					1.4	1.1

Denominator:

11 physicians x 275 days	=	3025 physician days
23 nurses/midwives x 275 days	=	6325 nurse days

5a)   bed occupancy $= \dfrac{16966}{77 \times 365} = 60.4\%$

As there seem to have existed some additional beds during the year ('number of available bed days'), we calculate

bed occupancy $= \dfrac{16966}{33289} = 51.0\%$

5b)   average length of stay $= \dfrac{16966}{2211} = 7.7$ days

6   There are only few and indirect quality indicators. Low institutional birth attendance. (If you calculate roughly that 4% of the population are pregnant women, i.e. 3700 in the district, only 15% of them have been attended by physicians and nurses and 11% by midwives. You get similar results if you take the number of registered births (3243).

Vaccination coverage is low (see below)

7.   (a) Coverage: 1932/3302   =   58.5%

        (b) intermittency of use: 5272/3708   =   1.4 (very low)

8.   No data about costs

9.   No data about the trend of morbidity and mortality rates.

        There is no equitable distribution of health posts and vaccination coverage among the different sub-districts. There is no data about risk groups.

Page 63   Equity

Equity can be assessed in terms of availability (i.e. are the existing resources equally available to the whole population?) and coverage (are the coverage rates for the different programmes equal for all groups of population, particularly for those at high risk, i.e. those who need it most?)

Page 81   Making a census

The possible solution to this exercise is threefold:

(a) The data on which the target is based is wrong

It is important to note that the target number of children under one year is taken from the census, which may or may not reflect the actual number of children. The estimates from the census (see below) may be too high or too low with respect to the real number of children under one year living in a given area. It is essential to discuss this with the local health workers so as to prevent feelings of frustration or undue pride.

(b) The health workers' unease of feeling controlled ('Perceived Threat Syndrome').

Health workers may perceive the graphic representation of their efforts as a threat, insofar as it testifies to their shortcomings and even their failures rather than to their unqualified accomplishment. They may then be unable to resist the temptation of presenting 'cooked' data. Here again, one should not lose sight of one of the basic premises of success for any given programme: good communication between supervisors and the local health personnel, which entails mutual trust as well as the willingness on the health workers' part to submit to necessary checks. And it should also be emphasized that achieving 100% coverage is not very likely owing to systematic deficiencies (which should be discussed in great detail) and to the inaccuracy of the existing data. You should make it very clear that the graphs are meant to show general tendencies that are liable to further interpretation. *(The supervisor must make every effort to find something encouraging to say referring to the local situation).*

(c) The wrong target

You should not set a target for every element in a programme. For instance, it would be a mistake to target the number of essential drugs to be taken per year by a given population. In doing so, you would contribute to the medicalization of the population.

Coverage: a measure, usually expressed as a percentage of people or households in need of a health service or facility who actually receive it, compared to all those who should receive it, e.g. households with a reasonably safe water supply, infant fully immunized with three doses of DPT vaccine (Vaughan and Morrow 1989).

APPENDIX B.3
DIDACTIC GAMES: OBJECTIVES, TARGETS AND INDICATORS

First Didactic Game: 'Talking to the neighbours'

Plan

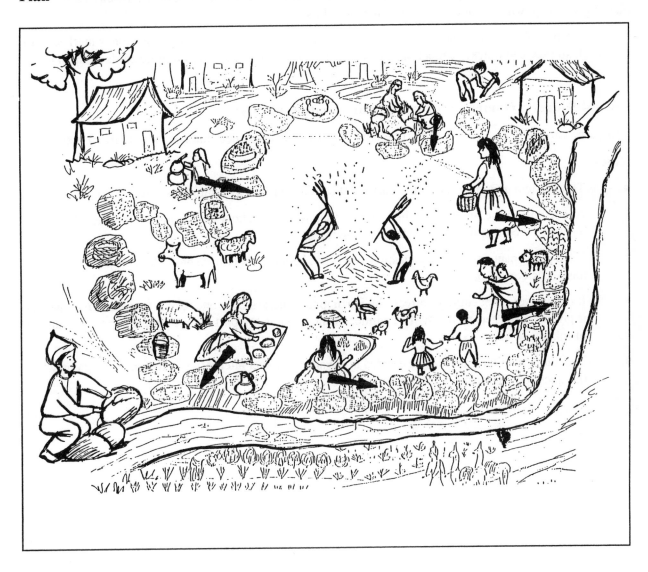

Rules

The map shows a rural community where women work in several types of activity. They want to go along the stoneway to be able to talk to each other.

Each player places a pawn on one of the women marked with an arrow. The first player throws the dice and moves along the stoneway as many stones as the dice says. If the stone reached has a symbol, the player has to take a card from the question bank, and must answer the question. If the answer is correct (according to the group's decision) the player receives two extra pawns; if the answer is only partially correct, the player gets one pawn; and none when the answer is false.

The other players follow the same rules. They can go both ways to be able to get on the stones marked with a symbol, so they can quickly collect pawns. The game ends when there are no more cards in the bank.

Second Didactic Game: 'Improving your shooting ability'

This game can have any number of participants, but it is recommended that not more than 10 play.

Rules

- The participants must throw the darts in the areas marked with numbers 1 to 3.

- According to the number reached, the participant must take a card from the question bank and answer the corresponding question (enumerated).

- If the participant answers the question correctly, he/she gets two tokens. The group decides if the answer is correct or not.

- If the answer is not entirely correct, the participant receives only one token; if an incorrect answer is given, he/she gets no token. The winner of the game is the participant with the greatest number of tokens.

- The duration of the game can be decided in advance. Another alternative is to finish the game when the question bank runs out of cards.

How to produce the darts

1. Take a piece of paper 15 x 15 cm; fold it as in fig. 2.

2. Take four matches and glue them between the folds of the paper. In the centre of the matches fix a pin (fig.3).

3. With a piece of thread, bind the four matches firmly.

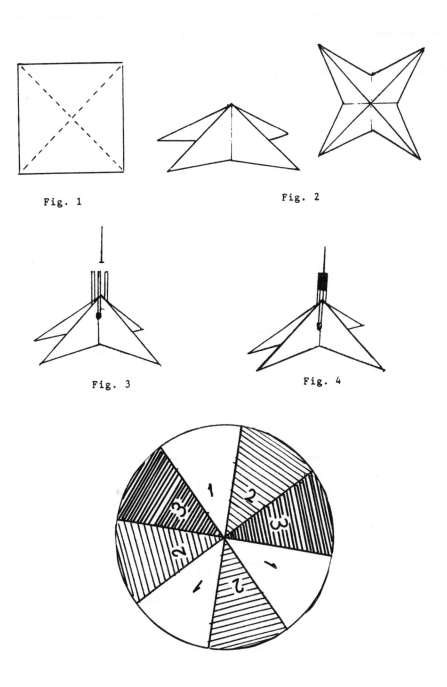

Fig. 1   Fig. 2

Fig. 3   Fig. 4

Question bank : (objectives, targets and indicators)

What does 'coverage' mean?	What is a 'target'?
What is the denominator of the availability indicator	What is the difficulty with accessibility indicators?
If a health programme is efficient, does it necessarily mean that it is effective?	How do you calculate the average length of a stay in hospital?
Which indicator is calculated by: $$\frac{\text{Vaccinated children}}{\text{children less than 1 year old}} \times 100?$$	Which indicators do you need in order to measure the input of a health service?
Name 3 examples of indicators of effectiveness	How do you evaluate the efficiency of a tuberculosis programme?
Does the efficiency of a health service provide information about its 'impact'?	What categories of accessibility to health services exist?
How do you calculate the extent of use of a service or programme?	How do you calculate the quality of a service or programme?

To what do the process indicators refer?

How do you calculate the percentage of occupied beds in a hospital?

To what category of indicators do
the following belong?
<u>No. of hours of vaccination personnel</u>?
       target population

To which indicator does the following belong?
<u>No. of days of occupied beds</u>
No. of days of available beds

How do you calculate birth attendance coverage?

How do you calculate vaccination coverage?

APPENDIX B.4
COMPARATIVE DATA FROM WORLD HEALTH STATISTICS[*]

AVAILABILITY

	No. physicians 10,000 inhabs.	No. nurses 10,000 inhabs.	No. hospital beds 1,000 inhabs.
Industrial countries			
USA/Canada*	21	82	6
Better-off developing countries			
Argentina	27	5	5
Uruguay*	19	5	5
Oman	9	25	2
Poor countries			
Peru*	10	8	2
Nicaragua*	7	4	2
Papua New Guinea	0.8	6	1
Very poor countries			
Bolivia	7	2	2
Haiti*	2	2	1
Ghana	0.8	6	1

PRODUCTIVITY

No. consultations/per health worker per day

Peru (South Andes)	5.1	(physicians; hospitals included)
Mexico (part of the	2.7	(physicians; hospitals included)
Federal District)	1.1	(auxiliary)

USE OF SERVICES

No. consultations/per inhabitant per year

Better–off developing countries

Mexico (North)	0.5	(rural areas)

Poor countries

Peru*	0.25	in the South Andes
	1.5	in the metropolitan area

---

*   Source: OPS, World Bank (1993)
Pabón 1985

155

IMMUNIZATION COVERAGE (UNICEF, 1986–87)

	% of children (<1 year) fully immunized with			
	DPT	Polio	Measles	BCG
Industrial countries				
USA	37	24	82*	not used
Better-off developing countries				
Argentina	75	85	81	91
Uruguay*	70	70	99	98
Mexico	62	97	54*	71
Tunisia	89	89	79	94
Poor countries				
Peru*	42	45	35	61
Nicaragua*	43	85	44	93
Zimbabwe	77	77	73	86
Very poor countries				
Bolivia	24	28	33	31
Haiti	20	28	23	45
Guinea	15	8	43	46
Benin	52	52	38	67
Nepal	46	40	22	78

---

*   1 — 5 years

EFFECTIVENESS (UNICEF 1987)

(Note: For the sake of brevity we present morbidity/mortality data for only one year. However, for the calculations of effectiveness the differences between different years should be used)

	Infant mortality rate	Mortality 1 – 4 years	Life expectancy at birth	% low birth weight
Industrial countries				
USA/Canada	10	13	76	7
Better-off developing countries				
Argentina	32	38	71	6
Uruguay	27	32	71	8
Mexico	48	70	69	15
Tunisia	60	86	66	7
Poor countries				
Peru	89	126	63	9
Nicaragua	63	99	64	15
Zimbwabwe	73	116	59	15
Very poor countries				
Bolivia	111	176	54	15
Haiti	118	174	55	17
Guinea	148	252	43	18
Benin	111	188	47	10
Nepal	129	200	52	10

APPENDIX B.5
EXERCISE ON THE USE OF INDICATORS

The Riverland district 1996 (real data)

Information about health services

Hospital

Personnel		
	10	Physicians
	3	Nurse-midwives
	16	Nurses
	1	Pharmacist technician
	25	Auxiliaries
	2	Nutritionist auxiliaries
	2	Laboratory auxiliaries
	42	Other technicians

Number of beds   77

Health centre

Personnel		
	1	Physician
	1	Nurse-midwife
	2	Nurses
	1	Pharmacist technician
	1	Auxiliary

Number of beds   0

11 Health posts

Personnel		
	1	Nurses
	14	Auxiliaries

Number of beds   0

Population in the District

Total	92,500
Births	3,243
<1 year	3,302
1-4 years	1,868
5-14 years	23,215
>14	64,115

Population in the District according to the health posts, health centres and data about vaccination doses in one year

Sub–district	Establishment	Population	<1 year	BCG	Measles	DPT III	Polio III
1. Checacupe	HP	5,710	194	188	135	196	196
	HP	720	24	252	119	193	193
2. Combapata	HP	4,900	167				
3. Marangani	HP	10,422	354	370	38	8	368
	HP	1,415	48				
4. Pitumarca	HP	6,024	205	265	201	370	197
5. San Pablo	HP	6,100	207	182	89	198	124
	HP	800	27				
6. San Pedro	HP	3,840	131	115	49	104	102
7. Sicuani	Hospital	48,138	1,637	1,850	1,166	1,323	1,324
8. Tinta	HP	6,030	205	183	135	159	159

Physicians = 250 vaccinations
Nurses = 292 vaccinations
Auxiliaries = the rest of vaccinations

Users and activities registered according to the health programmes

a) Programme	b) users	c) total activities	d) healthy	e) sick
00 Total	25,178	28,383	12,814	15,569
1.0 Maternal health	7,187	9,507	9,814	44
1.1 antenatal care	3,708	5,272	5,257	15
1.2 postnatal care	2,517	2,647	2,622	25
1.3 family planning	962	1,588	1,584	4
2.0 Child health	5,699	6,127	101	6,026
2.1 <1 year	1,853	1,966	33	1,933
2.2 1 – 4 years	2,222	2,386	18	2,368
2.3 5 years	292	322	7	315
2.4 6 – 14 years	1,332	1,453	43	1,410
3.0 Adult Health				
3.1 15–19 years	1,529	1, 579	502	1,077
3.2 20 years +	10,763	11,170	2,748	8,422

d) Activities by midwives and nurses

e) Activities by physicians

Consultation on out-patient clinic in family planning by midwives

Patient	total	Methods			
		IUD	pill	condom	other
0.0 New patients	962	253	289	334	85
1.0 Users	604	312	143	141	8
2.0 Non-attendees	18	18			
3.0 Complications	3	3			

Birth Attendance

Place	Physicians	Nurses	Midwives
Hospital	241	178	0
Home	9	144	407

Attendance by auxiliaries (in health post)

New patients   =   49, 926

Attendances   =   51, 088

Hospital (bed use statistics)

Number of admissions	=	2, 209
Number of discharges	=	2, 211
Alive	=	2, 113
Deaths	=	98
Number of occupied bed days	=	16, 966
Number of available bed days	=	33, 289
Live births	=	451
Foetal deaths and abortions	=	164 (24+140)

Assessment of health services by means of indicators

Answer the following questions (although in some cases there may be insufficient information).

1   **Accessibility**: what proportion of pregnant women can be brought to hospital by car within two hours, if severe problems arise during delivery?

(In each village assume that a car can be hired within one hour, in the case of an emergency)

What kind of information is necessary to answer this question?

2.   **Availability**: Calculate the availability of:

(a)   physicians, nurses and beds in the district.

3.   **Activities**:

(a)   what are the main activities of the physicians, nurses and auxiliaries?

(b)   which areas are weak?

4.   **Productivity**:

(a)   calculate the daily productivity of Health Posts, by physicians, nurses and midwives, taking into account that they are employed 6 hours per day, 275 days per year.

(b)   calculate the time they are spending per day on each of these activities, using the following table:

Type of activity	Total number of activities performed per year by		Total number of activities performed per day by		Minutes per day by	
	Physician	Midwives/ nurses	Physician	Midwives/ nurses	Physician	Midwives/ nurses
Consultations Weight monitoring Birth attendance Antenatal care Vaccination Family planning Adult monitoring Home visits						— 0.3 26.4 4.15 3.75 7.65 25.2 —
Total minutes Total hours						

Consultation in out-patient clinic	15 minutes
Adult monitoring	15 minutes
Weight monitoring	15 minutes
Birth attendance	120 min/doctor
	240 min/nurse-midwives
Antenatal care/postnatal care	10 minutes
Vaccination	5 minutes
Family planning advice	15 minutes
Home visits	90 minutes

5. **Utilization**

   (a)   calculate % bed occupancy

   (b)   calculate average length of stay

6. **Quality of cure and care**

   What information could you use as a proxy for the assessment of the quality of health services?

7. **Coverage**

   (a)   calculate the vaccination coverage with measles vaccines at the age of one year

   (b)   calculate the intensity of use of antenatal care

8. **Effectiveness**

   What measures of effectiveness can you find in the text?

9. Can you find examples of equity?

   Can you infer anything about risk groups or risk factors?

Additional questions:

- Is the data presented reliable?

- What possible biases might interfere?

BIBLIOGRAPHY

Alarcón, J. and A. Kroeger (eds),
   Taller Latinoamericano de Epidemiología Aplicada a los Servicios de Salud, 2nd edition, Lima, 1991.

Canales, F., E.L. Alvarado and E.B. Pineda,
   Metodología de la investigación, PAHO/WHO, Editorial Limusa, Mexico, 1986.

GTZ-ZOPP,
   An introduction to the method, Eschborn GTZ, Form 21–26, 3/87, 1987.

GTZ/ITHÖG,
   Indicators for district health systems (unpublished), Frankfurt–Heidelberg, 1990.

Kroeger, A. and R. Luna (eds),
   Atención Primera de Salud: Principios y Métodos, 2nd edition, Pax-Mexico, Organización Panamericana de la Salud, 1992.

Lutz, W.,
   Community Health Surveys. A practical guide for health workers, International Epidemiology Association, Switzerland, 1986.

McCusker, J.,
   How to measure and evaluate community health. A self-teaching manual for rural health workers, Macmillan Press, London and Basingstoke (First edition 1978 by AMREF), 1982.

McMahon, R., E. Barton, M. Pilot, N. Gelina and F. Ross,
   On being in charge: A guide to management in primary health care, WHO, Geneva, 1992.

Morley, D. and H. Lovel,
   My name is to-day: An illustrated discussion of child health, society and poverty in less developed countries. Macmillan Press, London and Basingstoke. 1986.

OPS,
   Desarrollo y forteleciemiento de los Sistemas Locales de Salud en la transformación de los sistemas nacionales de salud, Organización Panamericana de la Salud, Washington D.C., 1989.

Pabón, H.,
   Evaluación de los servicios de salud CEPADS, Universidad del Valle, Cali, Colombia, 1985.

Vaughan, J.P. and R.H. Morrow (eds),
   Manual of epidemiology for district health management, Special Programme for Research and Training in Tropical Diseases, WHO Geneva, 1989.

WHO,
   Making it work. Organisation and management of district health systems based on primary health care. WHO/SHS/88.1, Geneva, 1988.

WHO,
   The challenge of implementation. District health systems for primary health care, WHO/SHS/88.1., Rev.1, Geneva, 1988.